SURGICAL FINALS
Passing the Clinical
Second Edition

Gina R Kuperberg BSc MBBS(Hons), PhD
Assistant Professor, Harvard Medical School, Boston, USA.

John S P Lumley MS FRCS
Professor of Surgery, The University of London.
Honorary Consultant in Surgery,
St. Bartholomew's Hospital, London.
Council Member and Past Examiner in Anatomy
for the Royal College of Surgeons of England.

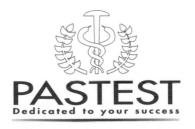

PASTEST
Dedicated to your success

First published 1996
Second edition 2003
Reprinted 2005

ISBN 1 901198 77 4

A catalogue record for this book is available from the British Library.

The information contained within this book was obtained by the authors from reliable sources. However, while every effort has been made to ensure its accuracy, no responsibility for loss, damage or injury occasioned to any person acting or refraining from action as a result of information contained herein can be accepted by the publishers or authors.

PasTest Revision Books and Intensive Courses
PasTest has been established in the field of postgraduate medical education since 1972, providing revision books and intensive study courses for doctors preparing for their professional examinations. Books and courses are available for the following specialities:
MRCP Parts 1 and 2, MRCPCH Parts 1 and 2, MRCS, MRCOG Parts 1 and 2, DRCOG, MRCGP, DCH, FRCA, PLAB, MRCPsych Parts 1 and 2.

For further details contact:
PasTest, Freepost, Knutsford, Cheshire WA16 7BR
Tel: 01565 752000   Fax: 01565 650264
Email: enquiries@pastest.co.uk   Web site: www.pastest.co.uk

Typeset by Saxon Graphics Ltd, Derby
Printed and bound in Great Britain by Bell and Bain Ltd, Glasgow

Contents

INTRODUCTION   vii

ACKNOWLEDGEMENTS   viii

PREFACE   ix

SYLLABUS CHECKLIST   x

COMPARISONS AND DIFFERENTIAL DIAGNOSIS   xiv

ABBREVIATIONS   xvi

SECTION 1- GENERAL POINTS
   1: The Clinical – format and preparation   3
   2: The Long Case/OSLER   7
   3: The Short Cases/OSCEs   11
   4: The Viva   15
   5: The day of the examination   21

SECTION 2 – HISTORY, EXAMINATION, TYPICAL CASES
   6: Pain, swellings and ulcers   25
   7: Neck swellings and thyroid lumps   41
   8: The breast   59
   9: The gastrointestinal tract   69
   10: The groin and scrotum   89
   11: Arterial insufficiency of the lower limb   105
   12: Venous disorders of the lower limb   117
   13: The hip   127
   14: The knee   137
   15: The hand and foot   151
   16: The post-operative patient   163
   17: General approaches   169

VIVA ANSWERS   173

RECOMMENDED READING LIST   197

REVISION INDEX   199

Introduction

By the end of clinical training, most students have accumulated enough knowledge to pass surgical finals. However, through poor organisation of the factual material, lack of confidence or examination stress, your performance may still be sub-optimal. This book is intended to reduce the chances of failure in the clinical part of the examination. It is not a comprehensive surgical text but provides relevant information for finals, particularly in the following areas:

- Useful tips for preparation of vivas, OSCEs, OSLERs and the long and short cases
- Relevant questions to include when taking a history in the long case
- Examination schemes designed to refine clinical skills
- Examples of typical cases, with lists of features, tables of differential diagnoses and common questions asked by examiners
- Popular viva questions at the end of each chapter and a separate answer section for self-assessment

The emphasis of this book is on a practical approach to clinical problems. The techniques described are applicable to the Final Examination and will keep your examiner happy. Additional checklists are provided to help you plan your revision. A concise, dogmatic and 'no-frills' approach has been taken to allow rapid retrieval and packaging of information, the aim at all times being to minimise your examination difficulties.

GK
JSPL

Acknowledgements

We thank Dr Mark Gurnell, and the many medical students who have read the text, for their helpful comments and suggestions. Also Helen Turner for battling with the tables and endless proof corrections in earlier drafts of the book.

GK would like to thank Michael Jacobson for his support and computer expertise. Most of all, she acknowledges the unfailing encouragement of her parents, Marcia and Louis Kuperberg, who have consistently taught her to see a project through from idea to completion.

Preface

The aim of this text remains to reduce the chances of failure in the clinical part of surgical finals. The core knowledge and skills needed to pass finals are those required to become a competent doctor and this final assessment should ensure that the student is fit for the practice of medicine. Over the last decade a number of new examination methods have emerged. This new edition addresses these developments and stands alongside its companion volumes of structured answers, OSCE and EMQ books. In the introduction to the long and short cases we consider how these traditional examination techniques relate to the newer OSLER and OSCE formats. In addition, we include brief notes on the investigation and treatment of the cases included throughout the book.

Finally, in response to student feedback, an additional chapter with the answers to the viva questions set at the end of each chapter is provided. We hope that the popularity of this book means that readers are passing their surgical finals; may this long continue.

Syllabus checklist

As an aid to revision, use this syllabus as your own personal checklist. Page numbers are given in brackets after each case. You should aim to achieve at least two ticks per case before the date of the examination. If you have not actually seen a condition, look it up in an illustrated textbook.

Read
Seen/Taught on
Happy with

Pain, swellings and ulcers
1. Squamous cell papilloma / Skin tag (30)
2. Wart (30)
3. Seborrhoeic keratosis / Senile wart (30)
4. Pigmented naevus or malignant melanoma (31)
5. Dermatofibroma / Histiocytoma (31)
6. Pyogenic granuloma (32)
7. Keloid or Hypertrophic scar (32)
8. Keratoacanthoma / Molluscum sebaceum (33)
9. Keratin horn (33)
10. Sebaceous cyst (33)
11. Boil or carbuncle (34)
12. Hydradenitis suppurativa (34)
13. Strawberry naevus (34)
14. Port wine stain (35)
15. Lipoma (35)
16. Dermoid cyst (35)
17. Ganglion (35)
18. Venous or traumatic ulcers (36)
19. Arterial–gummatous
         –neuropathic ulcers (37)
20. Basal cell or squamous cell carcinoma (38)

Neck swellings and thyroid lumps
1. Goitre (49)
2. Thyroglossal cyst (52)

	Read		
		Seen/Taught on	
			Happy with

3. Cervical lymphadenopathy (53)
4. Salivary Gland swelling (parotid and submandibular) (54)
5 Cervical rib (56)
6. Carotid body tumour (56)
7. Branchial cyst / sinus / fistula (56)

The breast
1. Breast carcinoma and Paget's disease of the nipple (63)
2. Fibroadenoma (65)
3. Fibroadenosis (66)
4. Nipple discharge (66)

The gastrointestinal tract
1. Hepatomegaly (78)
2. Splenomegaly (79)
3. Hepatosplenomegaly (80)
4. Enlarged kidneys (80)
5. Mass in right hypochondrium (82)
6. Mass in epigastrium (83)
7. Mass in left hypochondrium (83)
8. Mass in right loin (84)
9. Mass in umbilical region (84)
10. Mass in left loin (84)
11. Mass in right iliac fossa (84)
12. Mass in left iliac fossa (85)
13. Suprapubic mass (86)
14. Abdominal distension (87)

The groin and scrotum
1. Inguinal hernia (direct and indirect) (94)
2. Femoral hernia (97)
3. Saphena varix (99)
4. Femoral aneurysm (99)
5. Lymph nodes (99)
6. Psoas abscess (99)

Read

Seen/Taught on

Happy with

7. Testicular tumour (100)
8. Varicocoele (101)
9. Hydrocoele (101)
10. Epididymal cyst and spermatocoele (103)
11. Absent testis in a child (103)

Arterial insufficiency of the lower limb
1. Intermittent claudication (110)
2. Rest pain / critical ischaemia (114)
3. Diabetic foot (114)
4. Aortic aneurysm (115)
5. Amputation (115)

Venous disorders of the lower limb
1. Varicose veins (121)
2. Venous insufficiency (123)
3. AV malformations (124)

The hip
1. Hip pain (131)
2. Abnormal gait – antalgic and Trendelenburg (133)
3. Arthritis of the hip (134)

The knee
1. Knee pain (injuries and conditions in cases 2–6) (143)
2. Arthritides (osteorheumatoid and acute arthritis) (144)
3. Mechanical problems (meniscal tears, joint mice) (145)
4. Knee deformities (genu valgum and genu varum) (146)
5. Anterior knee swellings (prepatellar and infrapatellar bursae, Osgood-Schlatter's disease) (147)

	Read	Seen/Taught on	Happy with

6. Posterior knee swellings (semimembranous bursae, Baker's cyst, popliteal aneurysm, gout, tuberculosis) (148)

The hand and foot
1. Contracted hand (Dupuytren's and Volkmann's contractures, shortening of intrinsic muscles) (155)
2. Median nerve lesion (156)
3. Ulnar nerve palsy (157)
4. Radial nerve palsy (157)
5. Erb's palsy (157)
6. Klumpke's palsy (157)
7. Dropped finger (158)
8. Mallet finger (158)
9. Boutonnière's deformity (158)
10. Swan neck deformity (159)
11. Trigger finger / Stenosing tenosynovitis (159)
12. Rheumatoid arthritis (159)
13. Osteoarthritis (160)
14. The wasted hand (160)
15. Hallux valgus (bunions) (161)
16. Hammer toe (161)
17. Claw toes (161)

The post-operative patient (163)

Comparisons and differential diagnosis

Page numbers are given in brackets after each entry

Pain, swellings and ulcers
Hypertrophic scar vs keloid scar (32)
Furuncle vs carbuncle (34)
Ulcers: venous, arterial, traumatic, infective, neoplastic (36)
Ischaemic ulcer vs neuropathic ulcer (37)
Basal call carcinoma vs squamous cell carcinoma (38)

Neck swellings and thyroid lumps
Primary thyroid cancers: papillary, follicular, medullary, anaplastic malignant lymphoma (50)
Hyperthyroidism vs hypothyroidism (51)
Lateral neck swellings (52)
Cervical lymphadenopathy (53)
Mixed parotid tumour vs Warthin's tumour (55)
Midline neck swellings (49)
Causes of a goitre (49)
Salivary gland enlargement (54)
Features of malignancy of a parotid tumour (55)

The breast
Breast carcinoma, fibroadenoma, fibroadenosis (63)
Tethering vs fixation (64)
Differential diagnosis of breast carcinoma (64)
Paget's disease vs eczema (65)
Nipple discharge (67)

The gastrointestinal tract
Ileostomy vs colostomy (77)
Differential diagnosis of hepatomegaly (78)
Characteristics of an enlarged spleen (79)
Splenomegaly: massive, mild, moderate (79)
Characteristics of an enlarged kidney (80)
Enlarged left kidney vs enlarged spleen (81)

Characteristics of an enlarged gallbladder (82)
Masses: right loin, umbilical region, left loin (84)
Characteristics of a pelvic swelling (86)
Abdominal distension: fetus, flatus, faeces, fat, fluid (87)

The groin and scrotum
Direct hernia vs indirect hernia (97)
Inguinal hernia vs femoral hernia (97)
Inguinal swellings (99)
Scrotal and inguinoscrotal swellings (100)
Hydrocoele: vaginal, congenital, infantile, encysted hydrocoele of the cord (102)

Arterial insufficiency of the lower limb
Aorto-iliac vs femoro-distal disease (113)

Venous disorders of the lower limb
Superficial venous insufficiency vs deep venous insufficiency (123)

The hip
Hip pain (132)
Antalgic gait vs Trendelenburg gait (133)

The knee
Knee pathology vs referred pain (142)
Osteoarthritis vs rheumatoid arthritis (144)
Genu varum vs genu valgum (146)
Knee swellings (146)

The hand and foot
Causes of a contracted hand (155)
Finger deformities (158)
Characteristic deformities of rheumatoid arthritis (159)

Abbreviations

The following abbreviations have been used throughout this book

ASIS   anterior superior iliac spine
AV   arterio-venous
AXR   abdominal X-ray
CT   computerised tomography
CLL   chronic lymphocytic leukaemia
CXR   chest X-ray
DIP   distal interphalangeal
DVT   deep vein thrombosis
ECG   electrocardiogram
ENT   ear, nose and throat
FBC   full blood count
GIT   gastrointestinal tract
GP   general practitioner
HIV   human immunodeficiency virus
IP   interphalangeal
IVU   intravenous urogram
LFT   liver function tests
MCP   metacarpophalangeal
MRI   magnetic resonance imaging
PIP   proximal interphalangeal
PR   per rectum
T3   Triiodothyronine
T4   Thyroxin
TB   tuberculosis
TFT   thyroid function tests
TSH   Thyroid stimulating hormone
U&E   urea and electrolytes
UK   United Kingdom

Section 1
General points

1: The Clinical: examiners, patients and preparation

FORMAT

The examiners

Examiners traditionally work in pairs. There is normally one 'internal' examiner (from your own teaching hospital) and one 'external' (invited from outside).

You will usually be told who your examiners are. It is worth knowing their special interests, even though their questions may not be confined to these areas. Talk to medical students who have been taught by your examiners to find out individual preferences in examination technique (for example, always kneeling down to examine the abdomen).

The patients

The range of conditions you will see in the examination is not necessarily representative of the conditions seen in general hospital care. Firstly, you will never be given a very ill patient, with, for example, an acute abdomen or an acutely ischaemic limb. Secondly, there are some rare conditions which crop up disproportionately in examinations: such patients usually have long-standing problems with good physical signs. Examples are AV malformations or carotid body tumours.

Patients are drawn from four sources:

1. In-patients

Most in-patients transferred to the examination will be awaiting operations such as hernia repairs or removal of breast lumps. However, there is an increasing tendency to include post-operative patients in the clinicals: after all, you will be expected to manage such patients as surgical house officers. A minority of patients will be those recovering from acute conditions, with good histories and/or physical signs that have not yet resolved.

2. Patients coming up from clinics

Patients with good physical signs who attend clinics in the few weeks before the clinicals are often asked to come up for the examination. Try to attend clinics in your hospital in the lead-up to finals. (For example, prior to surgical finals, one of the authors walked into the examination centre with a fellow candidate who pointed out two patients she recognised: 'He has a sebaceous cyst on his forehead. She's got a left submandibular tumour'. After revising these two conditions, she was given both patients as short cases!)

3. 'Professional' patients

These are patients with long-standing signs who are listed on a computer data base and have been called up numerous times in the past. Such patients are usually excellent historians and may even point out their physical signs.

4. Simulated patients

Simulated patients are healthy individuals who are trained to simulate a patient's illness in a standard manner. They are usually actors. Some training is usually required to ensure that they are able to bring out the main points in the history on request and within the time allowed. Simulated patients can become skilled historians and very persuasive patients, such as when replicating a psychiatric disturbance. They are often asked to give their marks on the student encounter.

5. A video of a patient presenting a history

PREPARATION

Early preparation

Don't fall into bad habits

Ask a doctor to watch you examine and listen to your presentations as early and as often as possible. Without this, it is very easy to acquire bad habits that are difficult to break.

Act as a chaperone

Fourth-year medical students are often used as 'chaperones' in clinical examinations. Their role is to escort the candidates from room to room, ring the bells and ensure that the examination runs smoothly. If you are given this opportunity, take it. You will get an idea of the examination format and there will often be time to examine the patients yourselves afterwards. There can be no better preparation: some of the same patients may even come up the following year.

The revision period

1. Team up with a colleague

As the examination draws closer, pair up with a fellow student whose aims and standards are similar to your own and whose opinion you respect. By working in pairs, each of you can act as an examiner in turn, covering long and short cases and talking through topics that could arise in vivas. Remember that each person works at his/her own pace and thinks the other knows more than him/herself. The relationship should be mutually beneficial.

2. Ask for senior help

During the revision period, don't hesitate to ask for extra teaching from senior staff: they've all been through finals themselves and are usually glad to help. Don't be put off by the tendency to teach by humiliation and don't worry if you are given different information or conflicting approaches: just extract what you consider the best information from each teacher.

Bleep the house officer and ask for lists of patients to see as long and short cases. Ask when patients are to be admitted. Also find out when day surgery lists take place: here you will find many swellings, ulcers, varicose veins and hernias to examine.

3. Revise efficiently

This book gives plenty of lists of clinical features and provides tables of differential diagnoses. Modify these to make your own lists: you will remember best what you compile yourself. A card or computer system may be a useful revision aid at this stage.

Try not to work late into the night, relax before you go to bed, avoid excess coffee and keep up physical exercise. You will retain much more if you are alert during the revision period than if you are exhausted. Remember that hypnotics and anxiolytics may dull your mind on the day of the examination: take them only under medical supervision.

2: The Long Case/OSLER

Long cases in finals may be combined medical and surgical assessment with one or two examiners. You may or may not be observed during the history and examination. Often you are taken back to a patient to demonstrate specific signs.

The traditional long case format has inherent problems of objectivity and reliability. In response to such problems, there have been attempts to standardize patients and markings systems. These include the introduction of the "objective structured long examination record" (OSLER). The OSLER may include more than one case (a real patient, a simulated patient or a video, see page 4), each allocated 20-30 minutes, usually with a single examiner. This allows the examiner to test specific aspects of knowledge, skills or management decisions.

Allocating your time

Be sure you know well in advance how much time you will be given for the long case. This varies from school to school. Normally, twenty minutes is the minimum. This provides very little time for complex peripheral vascular or GIT problems. If it looks as if the history will take longer than half the allotted time, start examining after you have taken the details of presenting complaint and past medical history. The remainder of the history can be taken at convenient points during the examination. It is essential that you practise this.

Rapport with the patient

It is important to establish a good rapport with your patient. Be friendly and polite. Make sure the patient is comfortable at all times. Do not ask the diagnosis immediately. On the other hand, if you gain the patient's sympathy, he/she may point you in the right direction and may even show you physical signs.

The history

Go through your usual scheme which should by now be familiar. Start with name, age, occupation and marital status. This is followed by seven headings:

1. Presenting complaint

Ask about the main problem(s). List these together with a time scale, eg
* Abdominal pain: three weeks
* Nausea: four days

2. History of presenting complaint

Always include the systemic enquiry of the system relevant to the presenting complaint. Also ask the other appropriate questions (revised in sections of this book).

3. Past medical and surgical history

When asking about previous operations, remember to ask if there were any problems with the anaesthetic.

4. Drug history and allergies

5. Family history

Again, include questions about anaesthetic reactions.

6. Social history

A good social history will make you stand out from other candidates. Don't just ask about alcohol and smoking. It is important that you know how well the patient will manage at home during the post-operative period. Therefore ask about family, neighbours, carers, GP home visits, district nurses, home help, meals on wheels and financial problems.

Your social history should be relevant to the patient's problem. For example, if you have a patient with a stoma, enquire into the details of stoma care. If you have a patient with an orthopaedic problem or amputation, ask about physiotherapy, occupational therapy, aids and appliances.

7. Systemic enquiry

The examination

Start your examination by forming a general impression of the patient. Look for JACCOL (Jaundice, Anaemia, Cyanosis, Clubbing, Oedema, Lymphadenopathy). In your systems approach, pay particular attention to the system relevant to the presenting complaint. However, aim to be thorough: always take the pulse and blood pressure. Remember to test the urine. A dipstick should be provided.

Thinking time

You will usually have a few minutes between examining the patient and presenting your findings. During this time, reorganise any misplaced information and summarise the case in writing. You might also predict your examiners' questions so that you are one step ahead. The sections on 'typical cases' in this book will help you to do this.

Presenting your findings

The examiners will usually tell you what they want. Normally, they will ask you to tell them about the patient you have just seen. They may add a rider such as 'stick to the important features'. Don't get flustered if they start with 'What's the diagnosis?'.

If your patient was a poor historian, start by commenting on this fact: this is an important sign in itself and allowances will be made. However, it is no excuse for a poor presentation.

Your presentation should be as concise, snappy and comprehensive as possible. Place your notes in front of you for reference but talk, don't read, to the examiners. Don't panic if your notes are taken away from you: the history and examination will be fresh in your mind and you will remember more than you think.

If the patient has more than one complaint, this should be brought out by listing the presenting complaints. Then explain, 'I will describe each of these in turn'.

You should not give long lists of negative findings: if the main problem is abdominal and you have found no other abnormality, it is quite permissible to state 'other systems are normal'.

The examiners may interrupt you in the middle of your presentation. They may be happy with the way you have started and want to go on to the next point, they may wish to discuss a problem in more depth, or they may simply be bored after listening to several well-delivered histories in a row.

You may be taken back to the patient to demonstrate an abnormal finding. This does not necessarily mean that there is any doubt about your findings: you may have elicited a sign previously missed!

3: The Short Cases/OSCEs

Some medical schools have introduced the "objective structured clinical examination" (OSCE) to assess a broad range of knowledge and skills in a quantifiable valid and reliable form. The OSCE aims to assess your factual recall, your interpretative skills, your behavioural attitude in professional practice and your ability to perform particular practical tasks. It ensures that each of you is presented with the same material and therefore provides a uniform evaluation and marking system.

The OSCE often includes short cases. These are probably the most difficult part of the clinical examination as you will be required to examine a patient under the eagle eye of one or two examiners. The examiners will watch for three things:

A caring and competent approach

You should always introduce yourself. Fully expose the part of the body you wish to examine. Remember to compare both sides: if the examiner tells you to examine one leg, always expose the other as well. However, keep the patient 'decent'; for example, when exposing the legs, cover the groin. Before palpation, never forget to ask if there is any tenderness. The patient should be comfortable at all times. Thank the patient and cover him/her up before presenting your findings.

A good examination technique

Your examination of the short cases should be a smooth, thorough and a slick performance. The only way to achieve this is to practise again and again so that the routine becomes second nature.

Note the following points:

- Do not take the examination schemes provided in this book as gospel. Modify them according to your own teaching and individual preference.
- Don't be such an automaton that you fail to listen to the instruction: if the examiner tells you to 'palpate the abdomen', do not start with the hands.
- Passing the short cases is rather like passing a driving test: you must actually *show* your examiners that you are following the correct routine, for example by standing at the end of the bed to observe the patient.

- Although you are not supposed to take a history during the short case, you *are* allowed certain questions. For example, before examining a lump you cannot see, ask the patient to point out its exact position.

Three further questions that should be asked regarding a lump are: is it tender/painful (before you start)? How long have you had it? Is it changing in size?

There are certain parts that you are not expected to include in the examination situation, such as a rectal examination. However, you *must* indicate to the examiners that you would normally examine these areas. Furthermore you should express a desire to examine other systems to seek underlying causes of local conditions. For example, tell the examiners that you would like to examine the abdomen for secondary causes of hernias or varicose veins.

It is usually up to you whether you talk as you examine or present your findings at the end. Practise both ways: you may be requested specifically to 'explain what you are doing' or you may be interrupted at any stage of the examination to 'present your findings so far'.

An ability to elicit and draw conclusions from physical signs

You will not fail the examination if you do not pick up all the physical signs. However, you will be asked questions such as 'What are the causes of X?' and 'What is the differential diagnosis?'. Aim to be one step ahead of your examiners by pre-empting such questions.

Seek clues from the beginning: observe all the artefacts around the patient such as drips and catheters. Plastic gloves next to a patient with a submandibular swelling indicate that you are expected to palpate the gland bimanually. A glass of water next to a patient with a neck swelling suggests a goitre.

Never forget to look at the patient as a whole, even when you are asked to examine one small part: rheumatoid nodules on the elbow suggest the diagnosis before you have even looked at the hands.

Objective structured clinical examinations (OSCEs) have been designed to provide a broader coverage of knowledge and skills in a quantifiable, valid and reliable form. They aim to assess interpretive skills, as well as factual recall; they include task-oriented items and they can examine a candidate's powers of decision making and their behavioural attitude in simulated professional practice. The overall effect is to provide a more valid assessment of candidates for their subsequent clinical practice.

OSCEs bring a new dimension to the assessment of medical training. Of particular value is their ability to examine practical and other skills in a unified, measurable and reproducible fashion. This is in keeping with current trends towards performance based assessment throughout health care. OSCEs provide for an effective use of the examination time, examiners' time and commitment. They are effective in assessing knowledge and practical skills and ensure that each student is presented with the same material, thus providing a uniform evaluation with consistent marking of all those involved.

The preparation of OSCEs requires a good deal of thought and time. The whole staff should be aware of, and preferably involved in, their development and students should have experience prior to any examination so that they can be comfortable with this form of assessment. An OSCE requires a great deal of organization in collecting material, appropriate patients, laying out stations and making sure staff are available for manned areas. Setting up the examination can be costly on administration and on medical staff and patients, and includes the hidden costs of Faculty time in the development of the exercise.

Analysis of the data and ensuring the validity of the examination requires painstaking activity. The weighting of key questions on essential knowledge has to be resolved before any feedback to staff or students. Standard setting should be based on expected knowledge and the skills required and this relies as much on that much-criticized 'gut feeling' as it does on statistical formulae. Standardised patients, both actual and simulated have to be found and trained and an adequate pool must be available to cover expected needs. When introducing OSCEs, a school has to decide whether it is as an additional assessment or whether it should replace a previous part of the examination. If the latter, it is essential that other important areas are not diluted in the process. OSCEs are not ideal in assessing interpersonal skills: video clips or trained patients can be rather artificial in this respect. For patient examination, OSCEs do not provide a comprehensive evaluation of all aspects of a learning and educational programme and therefore should be part of a multi-component assessment in the final examination, forming a useful means of determining practical skills over a wide area.

In spite of their potential limitations, OSCEs do provide a valuable addition to the clinical exit examination and students and staff should become well acquainted with their format and appreciate their discriminatory properties.

4: The Viva

Vivas are still widely practiced in finals and postgraduate examinations. Although they can be subjective and provide a patchy assessment of the curriculum, they can cover essential knowledge in a form that relates to subsequent clinical practice. You may particularly dread it as the field is vast and 'they can ask you anything'. However, examiners usually follow fairly standard approaches and, by practising and paying due attention to viva technique, it should not be too much of an ordeal.

You should be aware that any part of the clinical examination may turn into a 'mini-viva'. Indeed, the sections of this book entitled 'typical cases' deal specifically with the types of questions asked as part of long and short cases.

VIVA TECHNIQUE

Note the following points:

- Go in with a positive attitude.
- Although you will be nervous, try not to show it: aim to give an impression of calm confidence.
- Try to hold the attention of your examiners: speak audibly and clearly. Keep eye contact with at least one of them.
- When asked a question, consider for a moment before rushing into an answer. However, do not hesitate too long as this makes you appear uncertain.
- If you do not understand a question, admit it, put it behind you and be ready for the next question.
- Once you get onto a topic you know, keep talking as long as you have positive factual knowledge to offer. Drop your voice slightly on the final sentence so the examiners know you have completed your statement: try not to peter out.
- Be confident in your knowledge: avoid words such as 'possible' and 'I think'. If an examiner says 'are you sure?', this does not necessarily mean that you are wrong. If, however, an examiner tells you that you are wrong, accept it, even if you are certain you are right. This is not the time for argument or confrontation.

- Don't dig yourself a hole by mentioning a very rare condition or something about which you know little or nothing. The examiner could very well ask you to elaborate ('Oh yes, tell me more about that').
- Don't worry if some humour arises and you are excluded: examiners are pleased to have some light relief during a heavy day's examining. However, do not go out of your way to be funny as this can fall very flat.
- At the end, do not rush off as soon as the bell rings: the examiner decides the finishing point, not you. When the end is signalled, smile and thank the examiners, regardless of your feelings. Leave quietly at a normal pace. Try not to trip, knock over the chair or slam the door!

ORGANISATION OF INFORMATION

Always show the examiners that you can classify information.

A disease

You may be asked to talk about a particular disease. Use a pathology sieve to structure your answer. One aide-memoir is 'Dressed In a Surgeon's Gown A Physician Might Make Progress': Definition, Incidence, Sex, Geography, Aetiology, Pathogenesis, Macroscopic pathology, Microscopic pathology, Prognosis. This can be slightly modified to form a clinical sieve '… a physician Should Succeed In Treatment': Symptoms, Signs, Investigations, Treatment.

Aetiology

Examiners often ask the causes of a condition. Remember to mention common causes before rarer ones. If you have not memorised a list for that condition, again refer to a sieve. You may find the following mnemonic useful: CIMETIDINE: Congenital, Infective, Inflammatory, Metabolic, Endocrine, Traumatic, Iatrogenic, Degenerative, Idiopathic, Neoplastic, Everything else!

Management

The question 'How would you manage a patient with this condition?' comes up again and again. The term management is sometimes used loosely to be synonymous with treatment. However, management refers to history, examination, special investigations *and* treatment. You should *always* begin by saying 'I would take a thorough history and perform a full examination'. Go on to describe the special investigations you would request and only then describe the treatment. If asked about the management of trauma or shock, never forget to say: 'This is an emergency. I would first check the airway, the breathing and the circulation'.

Special investigations

When asked about special investigations, start with simple investigations such as urinalysis and blood tests: haematological (FBC, clotting studies, group and save) and biochemical (U&E, LFTs, TFTs, amylase). Then go on to describe relevant imaging investigations (CXR, ultrasound and Doppler's, angiography, barium studies, CT and MRI scans) and biopsies (cytology and histology). Remember that all older patients being considered for surgery should have a CXR and ECG.

Treatment

If asked about the treatment of any disease, always divide your answer into conservative, medical and surgical. Under conservative treatment, consider the contributions from all other providers such as nurses, physiotherapists, occupational therapists and social services. Under medical treatment, consider drugs, chemotherapy and radiotherapy.

TOPICS COVERED IN VIVAS

Objects used as talking points

Examiners will often have an array of objects in front of them which serve as useful talking points.

Results of investigations

Familiarise yourself with AXRs, barium studies, IVUs and angiograms. Examiners like to know if you have actually seen these investigations and may ask you to describe the procedures. You should also know normal haematological and biochemical values.

Pathology specimens

If handed a pathology pot, start by noting the organ. Then describe the abnormalities and make a diagnosis. Look all around the specimen: a discouraging amorphous mass on one view may be easily recognised by the presence of a nipple or an appendix on the other side. You may then be asked about the condition and how the patient presented.

Other objects

You are expected to recognise a variety of instruments and tubing. These include an endotracheal tube, a laryngoscope, a Guedel airway, a laryngeal mask, a chest drain, a tracheostomy tube, a Sengstaken-Blakemore tube, a T-tube, a proctoscope and a sigmoidoscope. You may be asked to describe a practical procedure such as how to catheterise or how to put down an endotracheal tube.

Other popular viva topics

Popular viva questions are listed at the end of each chapter in this book. You should be particularly aware of the following topics:

Emergencies

You must know about the management of the common surgical emergencies such as the acute abdomen and acute upper and lower GI bleeding. These are 'Pass/fail' questions.

Anatomy and embryology

You are not expected to know much anatomy, embryology or details of operations. However, there are certain topics which are particularly popular with examiners. These include the anatomy of the inguinal and femoral canals, tracheostomy sites and the embryology of thyroglossal and branchial cysts.

General surgical care

It is essential that you know about fluid balance, post-operative complications and complications of fractures.

Topical questions

Keep an eye out for topical issues raised in the media and try to read the leaders of the *Lancet* or *British Medical Journal*.

5: The day of the examination

The examination week is very intensive. Each day covers long cases/OSLERs and short cases/OSCEs, plus one or more vivas. It therefore deserves fore-thought and preparation, particularly on what you intend to take with you, what you will wear and how you will make your way to the examination.

Take appropriate equipment

Work out in advance exactly what you intend to carry. Know what equipment is in which pocket. Bring the following items:

- Watch with a second hand
- Stethoscope
- Short ruler
- Tape measure
- Pen torch (plus extra batteries)
- Opaque tube, eg an empty Smartie tube (for transillumination)
- Wooden spatulae (for looking in the mouth)
- Tourniquet (for examining varicose veins)

Neurological examination requires additional items which you can bring yourself. However, they will usually be provided.

- Cotton wool
- Sterile, sheathed disposable needles
- Tuning fork
- Tendon hammer
- Orange sticks (for eliciting plantar responses)
- Red- and white-headed hat pins (each > 5 mm diameter)
- Pocket-sized reading chart
- Ophthalmoscope

Dress conventionally

Avoid appearing at all unconventional. Men should wear a plain dark suit, tie and white shirt. Women should wear a smart dress or suit. Hair should be tidy: men should have a recent haircut and women with long hair should tie it back. Make sure your nails are clean and your shoes polished.

Arrive on time

It is essential that you arrive on time and in a composed state. You can be sure that there will be examiners and patients waiting for you, regardless of traffic delays or train strikes. Excuses wear thin on such occasions. If you are not familiar with the venue, a preliminary visit may be worthwhile in order to time your journey.

Aim to be at the examination at least thirty minutes before the listed starting time. This will ensure you are able to find the toilets, check your dress and equipment, and fill in any necessary forms. It is a good idea, whilst waiting outside the examination room, to write down the various headings of your history and examination on the blank paper provided. Not only does this ensure you do not forget a heading in the heat of the situation, but it limits the space (and hence time) that you spend on any one area.

Section 2
History, examination, typical cases

6: Pain, swellings and ulcers

THE HISTORY

Pain, swellings and ulcers are presenting features of many diseases. Always ask the same questions:

Pain

- Where is the pain? (Ask the patient to point to the area where the pain is felt maximally)
- Have you ever had a pain like this before?
- When did you first notice the pain this time?
- Did the pain begin suddenly or gradually?
- Has the pain become worse since it started?
- Can you describe the pain? (?colicky ?burning ?aching)
- How severe is the pain? Does it keep you awake at night
- Does the pain go anywhere else?
- Is there anything that makes the pain better?
- Is there anything that makes the pain worse?
- What do you think caused the pain?

A mnemonic may help you remember the important features: **S**ite, **R**adiation, **S**everity, **N**ature, **O**nset, **P**eriodicity, **D**uration, **R**elieved by, **A**ccentuated by, **T**iming, (eg **S**tate **R**egistered **S**taff **N**urse; **O**ut **P**atients **D**epartment; **RAT**).

A swelling or an ulcer

- When did you first notice it?
- How did you notice it?
- Has it changed since you first noticed it?
- Has it ever completely disappeared since you noticed it?
- How does it bother you? (What are the main symptoms: is it painful or tender?)
- Do you have (or have you ever had) any other lumps or ulcers?
- What do you think caused it?

25

THE EXAMINATION

Even if the diagnosis seems obvious, always go through the same routine when examining a swelling or an ulcer. It is probably easier to talk as you go rather than to present your findings at the end.

'Examine this patient's swelling'

ACTION	NOTE
Introduce yourself	
Ask permission to examine the patient	
Expose the lump completely	
LOOK	
Inspect the lump	*?shape* *?colour*
Measure: • distance from the nearest bony prominence • dimensions	*?position* *?size*
FEEL	
Ask if the lump is tender/painful	Note if any part is sensitive on subsequent palpation
a. Temperature Run the backs of your fingers over the surface and surrounding area	*?warm*
b. Surface Feel with the pulps of your fingers	*?smooth* *?bosselated* *?rough*

c. Edge
Feel with your finger and thumb | *?clearly/poorly defined*

d. Consistency | *?stony-hard*
?rubbery-hard
?spongy
?soft

e. Surrounding area | *?indurated*

PRESS

a. Pulsatility
Rest a finger of each | *?expansile pulsation* (fingers
hand on opposite sides | pushed apart)
of the lump for a few seconds | *?transmitted pulsation* (fingers
Watch your fingers | pushed in same direction)

b. Compressibility/ reducibility
Press the lump firmly | *?compressible*
and then release the | (lump disappears on pressure and
pressure | reappears on release)
| *?reducible*
| (lump reappears only on
| application of another force, eg
| coughing, gravity)

c. Percussion
Percuss over lump | *?dull*
| *?resonant*

d. Fluctuation/fluid thrill
Place two fingers of one | Use this test for a *small* lump
hand at opposite ends of
the lump

Press the middle of the | *?fluctuant*
lump with the index | (two fingers move apart when
finger of your other hand | middle area pressed)

Repeat in a perpendicular plane

Ask patient to place the edge of his/her hand in the middle of the swelling
Flick on one side and feel on other side for a percussion wave

Use this test for a *large* swelling

?fluid thrill

MOVE

Try to move the skin over the lump

?fixation to skin
(skin cannot be moved over lump)

Try to move the lump in two planes at right angles to each other

?mobility

Ask patient to tense the underlying muscle
Reassess mobility

?attachment to underlying muscle
(movement *reduced* when underlying muscle tensed or 'disappears' beneath it)

LISTEN

Auscultate over the lump

?bruit
?bowel sounds

TRANSILLUMINATE

Press a pen torch and an opaque tube (eg a Smartie tube) on opposite sides of the lump
Look down the opaque tube

?transilluminable
(transillumination can only be accurately assessed by looking down the opaque tube)

EXAMINE SURROUNDING TISSUES

Examine regional lymph nodes:
• limbs/trunk–axillary nodes
• head/neck–cervical nodes

?local lymphadenopathy

Test sensation in the surrounding area

?local neurological deficit

Test the power of related muscles

?weakness

'Examine this patient's ulcer'

ACTION	NOTE	
LOOK		
Measure:		
● distance from the nearest bony prominence	*?position*	
● dimensions	*?size*	
	?shape	
Inspect the base	colour:	*?red/granulation tissue*
	penetration:	*?tendon*
		?bone
	discharge:	*?blood*
		?pus
Inspect the edge	edge:	*?flat sloping:*
		?punched out:
		?undermined:
		?raised:
		?raised and everted:
Measure the depth in mm	*?depth*	
FEEL		
Ask if the surrounding area is tender		
Feel with the backs of your fingers	*?warm*	

EXAMINE SURROUNDING TISSUES

Examine the regional lymph nodes	?*local lymphadenopathy*
Test sensation in the surrounding area	?*local neurological deficit*
Test the power of related muscles	

TYPICAL CASES

1. LUMPS AND SWELLINGS

Neck, breast, abdomen and knee swellings are covered on pages 49–57, 63–67, 76–87, and 142–148. This section revises skin lumps, giving examples of common short cases.

Lesions derived from the epidermis

Case 1: Squamous cell papilloma / Skin tag

This is a pedunculated overgrowth of skin. It is soft, the colour of normal skin and may occur at any site.

Treatment: Excision if symptoms, tying base where possible.

Case 2: Wart

Warts are grey/brown filiform lesions, usually seen on the back of the hand. The surface is rough and the consistency, hard.

Treatment: If symptoms paint podophyllin, freeze or curettage.

Case 3: Seborrhoeic keratosis / Senile wart

These are flattened, well-defined plaques, usually found on the back. They may be multiple and are usually pigmented. The patient will probably be elderly. They are easily recognised because of their greasy, rough surface and because they are easy to pick off (although you should not try to do this if you are uncertain of the diagnosis).

Case 4: Pigmented naevus or malignant melanoma

Benign naevi may occur anywhere. They may be flat, raised, hairy or non-hairy. The surface may be rough or smooth.
You should know the characteristics that suggest malignancy:

- Increase in size
- Ulceration
- Change in colour
- Irritation
- Bleeding
- Halo of pigmentation
- Satellite nodules
- Enlarged local lymph nodes
- Evidence of distant spread

Treatment:

- Benign – excise if symptoms
- Malignant – confirm diagnosis by excision or biopsy. Aim to eradicate by wide local excision and nodes. Cytotoxic drugs and radiotherapy for palliation.

Note: squamous cell and basal cell carcinomas may also present as epidermal nodules. They usually ulcerate and are considered in section 2, page 38.

Lesions derived from the dermis

Case 5: Dermatofibroma / Histiocytoma

This is a firm nodule, usually seen on the lower leg. It is part of the skin and fully mobile.

Treatment: Excise if symptoms.

Case 6: Pyogenic granuloma

This is a bright-red or blood-encrusted nodule. It feels fleshy and is slightly compressible. It bleeds easily.

If you are not sure of the diagnosis, ask the patient how quickly it appeared (it arises within days) and whether he/she remembers a preceding penetrating injury.

Note: unlike its name implies, it is not granulomatous or pyogenic. It is actually an acquired haemangioma.

Treatment: Excision.

Case 7: Keloid scar or Hypertrophic scars

Keloid is an overgrowth of fibrous tissue within a scar. Suspect this in a Black patient who has had a recent operation.

You may be asked about the differences between a keloid and a hypertrophic scar:

	HYPERTROPHIC SCAR	KELOID SCAR
Overall incidence	More common	Less common
Association with race?	No	Yes: more common in Afro-Caribbean people
Extent of overgrowth	Confined to scar tissue	Extends into surrounding tissue
Resolves spontaneously?	Yes: within a few months	No
Recurs after surgery?	No	Yes

Treatment: Leave six months to mature. Do not excise – recurs. Inject triamcinolone.

Lesions derived from skin appendages

Case 8: Keratoacanthoma / Molluscum sebaceum

A keratoacanthoma is a benign overgrowth of a sebaceous gland.

It appears within three to four weeks. It resembles a volcano, consisting of a conical lump of normal skin colour with a central crater containing keratin.

It usually regresses spontaneously but may take six to nine months.

Treatment: Only excise if diagnosis is uncertain or marked symptoms.

Case 9: Keratin horn

This is a dry, hard spike, derived from sebaceous secretions. Unlike a keratoacanthoma, it does not regress.

Treatment: Excise if symptoms.

Case 10: Sebaceous cyst

This is an extremely common short case. It is usually found in hairy areas (the scalp, neck, face and scrotum).

The size varies but the lump is usually hemispherical with a well-defined edge. Although it lies subcutaneously, it is attached to skin by the sebaceous duct.

The *consistency* is hard although there is some fluctuation. It is not usually transilluminable.

Always look for a punctum: only 50% will possess one but it is pathognomonic if you find it.

If the cyst is painful and red, this does not necessarily indicate infection: following trauma, the secretions may cause a foreign body inflammatory response in the surrounding tissues. Bacteria, however, cannot usually be cultured.

If you are asked about its origin, remember that the term 'sebaceous' cyst is a misnomer. It is **not** derived from the sebaceous gland, but from the outer sheath of the hair follicle. The cyst contents, although thick and waxy, are dead epithelial elements rather than sebaceous secretions.

Treatment: Excision, antibiotics for cellulites, drain abscess.

Case 11: Boil or carbuncle

A boil or furuncle is an infection originating in a hair follicle. It begins as a hard, red tender lesion. It later discharges spontaneously.

If you are allowed to ask the patient a few questions, ask about diabetes, steroid therapy and other predisposing immunodeficiencies.

You may be asked to describe the differences between a furuncle and a carbuncle:

	FURUNCLE	CARBUNCLE
Site	Skin	Subcutaneous tissue
Number of abscesses seen	One	Several
Appearance	Discrete lesion	Generalised necrotic area

Treatment: Wait for resolution unless cellulites (antibiotic) or abscess (drain).

Case 12: Hydradenitis suppurativa

A red, tender swelling is not necessarily a boil: if the patient has *multiple* such lesions in the *axillae* or *groin*, suspect hydradenitis suppurativa – infection of sweat glands.

Treatment: Antiobiotics, drain abscess. Wide excision recurrent problems.

Lesions derived from vascular structures

The term 'haemangioma' encompasses many lesions, including Campbell de Morgan spots and spider naevi.

You should also be able to recognise the two common paediatric haemangiomata.

Case 13: Strawberry naevus

This is a bright-red, strawberry-like lesion. It is small at birth but increases in size and may be disfiguring.

Treatment: It should be left alone, as it spontaneously regresses by the age of about four to five years. Remember the important exception to this rule is when it obscures a visual field.

Case 14. Port wine stain

As its name implies, this is a flat purple/red lesion with an irregular border. It is present at birth and does not increase or decrease in size thereafter.

Treatment: Cosmetic creams; excise or inject symptomatic varices and redundant skin.

Lesions not attached to skin

Case 15: Lipoma

This is a benign tumour of adipocytes. Its size varies. The *shape* is hemispherical and the *edge* is well-defined. The *consistency* is soft and the *surface*, bosselated.

Note: only **large** lipomas are fluctuant and transilluminable.

Lipomas are usually freely mobile although they may occasionally lie beneath the deep fascia.

Treatment: Excision.

Case 16: Dermoid cyst

Dermoid cysts are hard and spherical. Although derived from epithelial elements within the dermis, they lie subcutaneously.

In an adult, you should suspect an *implantation* dermoid, usually found on the fingers. Ask about a preceding injury.

In a child, suspect a *congenital* dermoid. This occurs at the sites of fusion of the facial processes, eg the outer angle of the eye.

Treatment: Excision.

Case 17: Ganglion

The patient will have a smooth, hemispherical swelling near a joint or tendon. The most common sites are at the wrist, on the dorsum of the hand and around the ankle. The *surface* is smooth and the *consistency*, firm. It is slightly fluctuant and weakly transilluminable.

Remember to palpate the ganglion in all positions of the underlying joint: its mobility depends on whether it is derived from, and thus attached to, deep structures.

35

Note that the origin is controversial. Some view it as a pocket of synovium, communicating with the associated joint. Others see it as a myxomatous degeneration of fibrous tissue, derived from the tendon sheath.

Treatment: Excision.

2. ULCERS

You should know the definition of an ulcer: a defect in an epithelial surface. You may be asked the causes:

TYPE	CAUSE	UNDERLYING DISEASE
Venous (page 122) (75% of leg ulcers)	(i) *Superficial venous insufficiency* (ii) *Deep venous insufficiency*	● Varicose veins ● Previous DVT
Arterial (page 114)	(i) *Large vessel disease (ischaemic)*	● Atheroma ● Beurger's disease
	(ii) *Small vessel disease (vasculitis)*	● Rheumatoid arthritis ● Polyarteritis nodosa
Traumatic	(i) *Neuropathic/trophic*	● Alcohol ● Diabetes mellitus ● Tabes dorsalis ● Syringomyelia
	(ii) *Others*	● Bedsores ● Self-inflicted injury
Infective	*Often associated with malnutrition*	● Pyogenic organisms ● Tertiary syphilis ● Mycobacterium ulcerans
Neoplastic	(i) *Primary neoplasm*	● Squamous cell carcinoma ● Basal cell carcinoma ● Malignant melanoma
	(ii) *Secondary neoplasm*	

Case 18: Ulcer with a sloping edge

A sloping edge is characteristic of a *healing* ulcer, ie a *traumatic* (although not neuropathic) ulcer or a *venous* ulcer.

Venous ulcers are found in the 'gaiter area' (above the malleoli, particularly the medial malleolus). They are usually shallow and flat. The base is covered with pink granulation tissue mixed with white fibrous tissue.

Look for and describe associated signs of superficial or deep venous insufficiency (see page 123).

Case 19: Ulcer with a 'punched-out' edge

It is unlikely that you will see a gumma of tertiary syphilis which is the classic 'punched-out' ulcer. This usually occurs on the anterior aspect of the lower leg and is easily recognised by the yellow-coloured ('wash-leather') base. Ischaemic and neuropathic ulcers are much more common short cases. They have many of the same characteristics:

- Over the tips and between toes
- Over pressure areas (heel, malleoli)
- Pale pink base (very little granulation tissue)
- Deeply penetrating
- Bone, ligaments and tendons seen in the base

Ischaemic ulcers are secondary to circulatory insufficiency (large or small vessel disease) whereas *neuropathic ulcers* are usually secondary to spinal cord disease or a peripheral neuropathy: repeated injury arises from loss of pain. Remember that diabetes mellitus has a *mixed* pathogenesis (see page 114).

If you are asked to distinguish between the two, use the following scheme:

	ISCHAEMIC ULCER	NEUROPATHIC ULCER
Ask if the ulcer is painful	Painful	Painless
Look for associated black eschar	Present	Absent
Feel the temperature of the surrounding area	Cold	Warm
Test the sensation of the surrounding area	Sensation intact	Sensation lost

Case 20: Ulcer with a raised edge

Ulcers with raised edges are neoplastic. The centre of the carcinoma becomes necrotic, but the periphery continues to grow and rises above the surface of the surrounding skin.

The main features distinguishing a basal cell carcinoma (rodent ulcer) from a squamous cell carcinoma are the *edge* and the *colour*:

	BASAL CELL CARCINOMA	SQUAMOUS CELL CARCINOMA
Edge	Raised	Raised and everted
Colour	Pearly, glistening, pink tinge (due to fine telangiectasia)	Red-brown (due to vascularity)

You should be able to list the predisposing factors for skin cancer:

- Age
- Sunlight (ultraviolet radiation)
- Ionising radiation
- Chemical irritants (eg soot, dyes, tar)

Remember that malignant change (usually to squamous cell carcinoma) may also occur in long-standing benign ulcers (Marjolin's ulcers), in scars and in chronically discharging osteomyelitis sinuses.

Treatment of ulcers: Make diagnosis

Venous – four-layer compression bandaging.

Neuropathic – daily inspection of feet, protect against trauma, clean and bandage.

Arterial – improve blood supply, may need amputation.

Infective – treat cause, antibiotics for cellulitis, drain abscesses.

Malignant – excise with nodes, chemotherapy and radiotherapy palliation.

Non-malignant – skin graft, persistent ulcers once granulated base.

POPULAR VIVA QUESTIONS

1. Describe the features you would note in examining a lump/an ulcer. How would these features help in your differential diagnosis?

2. What is the difference between a furuncle and a carbuncle?

3. What are the differences between a keloid and a hypertrophic scar?

4. What are the features that would suggest malignancy in a pigmented naevus?

5. Describe the differences in appearance between a basal cell carcinoma and a squamous cell carcinoma.

6. What aetiological factors may predispose to squamous cell carcinoma?

Answers on page 173

7: Neck swellings and thyroid lumps

THE HISTORY

If your patient complains of a swelling in the neck, ask the same questions as for any lump (page 25).

If you suspect lymphadenopathy, ask the following questions to determine local causes:

- Do you have any mouth ulcers or pain in your mouth?
- Do you have any pain or discharge from your nose or ears? – Do you have a sore throat?
- Have you noticed any other lumps on your head or face? – Do you have any difficulty swallowing?
- Do you have any difficulty breathing?

Your systemic enquiry will be important in determining *generalised* causes. If you suspect a goitre, ask the following specific questions:

Local effects of the swelling

- Is the lump painful?
- Do you have any difficulty or pain when you swallow?
- Do you have any difficulty breathing?
- Have you noticed any change in your voice recently?

Eye problems associated with hyperthyroidism

- Do you have double vision?
- Do you get painful, red eyes?

Systemic enquiry to determine thyroid status

1. General symptoms

- Have you noticed a change in your appearance?
- Are you intolerant of hot or cold temperatures?

2. Gastrointestinal symptoms

- Have you noticed a change in your appetite/weight/bowel habit?

3. Cardiorespiratory symptoms

- Do you get palpitations/shortness of breath on exertion/ankle swelling/ chest pain?

4. Neurological symptoms

- Have you noticed any nervousness/irritability/insomnia/loss of concentration?

5. Gynaecological symptoms (in females)

- Have you noticed any change in your menstrual cycle?

THE EXAMINATION

A common instruction in the short case is to 'examine this patient's neck' without being given any clue as to the pathology. Alternatively, you may be asked to 'examine this patient's thyroid gland'. In this case, proceed to the relevant section of the examination scheme below. Rarely, you may be pointed out a lump and asked to describe it (pages 26–28).

The presence of a glass of water near the patient is a good hint that there may be a goitre!

Always describe the position of neck swellings in terms of the triangles of the neck:

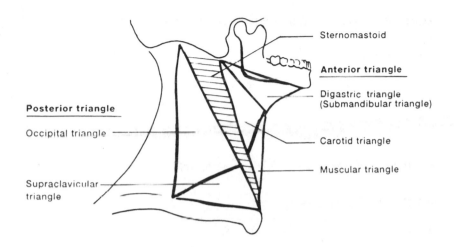

'Examine this patient's neck'

ACTION	NOTE
Introduce yourself	
Ask permission to examine the patient	
Expose the neck, with the patient sitting up comfortably	
LOOK	
Observe from in front and from either side	?*hyperaemia of skin* ?*scars* ?*distended neck veins* ?*obvious goitre* (between thyroid cartilage and manubrium sterni)
Ask patient to take a sip of water and to hold it in his/her mouth Then ask patient to swallow	?*goitre* (moves on swallowing)
Ask patient to stick out tongue	?*thyroglossal cyst* (moves up when tongue stuck out)

NOW PROCEED AS FOLLOWS:
- If *obvious goitre*, continue examination of thyroid gland: A (below)
- If *no goitre*, examine for cervical lymphadenopathy: B (page 46)
- If you *feel an obvious lump*, proceed to C (page 47)
- If you *suspect enlargement of a salivary gland*, proceed to D (page 48)

A. Examination of thyroid gland

ACTION	NOTE
LOOK (see previous page)	
FEEL	
Stand behind patient	
Ask if the swelling is tender	
Feel with the flat of your fingers over the thyroid (thumbs posteriorly)	
Tell patient to take another sip of water, to hold it in his/her mouth and then to swallow	*?thyroid felt to move on swallowing*
Palpate gently	*?tender* *?diffusely enlarged swelling* *?single nodule* *?multi nodular goitre* *?texture* *?surface* *?approximate size*
Palpate the cervical lymph nodes	*?associated lymphadenopathy* (page 46)
Whilst still standing behind patient, look over the top of his/her head	*?exophthalmos*

ASSESS POSITION

Stand in front of patient

Palpate the trachea in the suprasternal notch	*?trachea deviated*
Percuss the thyroid	*?lower limit of retrosternal extension*
Auscultate over the thyroid	*?bruit*

ASSESS THYROID FUNCTION

a. Observe overall
Look at patient's:
- face and skin — *?dry/shiny skin*
- build — *?thin/fat*
- dress — *?appropriate for temperature*
- behaviour — *?agitated/lethargic*

b. Examine the hands
Look at:
- palms — *?palmar erythema*
- nails — *?thyroid acropachy*

Feel:
- palms — *?sweaty*
- pulse — *?large volume*
  ?atrial fibrillation

Ask patient to hold arms outstretched — *?fast postural tremor*

c. Examine the eyes
Look at:
- conjunctiva — *?chemosis/oedema/redness*
- relationship of eyelid to iris — *?lid retraction*

Ask patient to follow your finger up and down — *?lid lag*

Test the eye movements:
- Ask patient to follow a
white hat pin with eyes
- Ask him/her to report any   *?ophthalmoplegia*
double vision

d. Assess neurologically
Ask patient to rise from a   *?proximal myopathy*
squatting position (or chair)   (a sensitive indicator of
without using hands for support   hypo/hyperthyroidism)

Test reflexes, observing the   *?slow-relaxing reflexes*
relaxation phase: (suggests hypothyroidism)
- supinator
- biceps

B. Examination for cervical lymphadenopathy

ACTION   NOTE

Stand behind patient
Examine lymph nodes
systematically:

First feel the horizontal ring:
- submental
- submandibular
- pre-auricular
- post-auricular
- occipital

Then feel the vertical chain: *?position of enlarged nodes*
- deep cervical
- posterior triangle
- supraclavicular

If you feel enlarged cervical
lymph nodes,

Look in the mouth, ears and   *?primary site of infection*
throat with pen-torch   *?primary malignancy*

Say you would request a full
ENT examination

Look carefully at the face and all
over the scalp

Examine:
- inguinal nodes
- axillary nodes
- epitrochlear nodes

?generalised lymphadenopathy

Examine patient above the
umbilicus

?skin lumps
?normal respiratory system
?breast lumps   ·

Examine the abdomen

?splenomegaly ?hepatomegaly

C. Examination of other neck lumps

ACTION	NOTE
Assess as for any lump (pages 26–28)	*?neck triangle* *?shape* *?colour* *?size* *?temperature* *?surface* *?edge* *?consistency*
Palpate lump as patient contracts the underlying muscle: eg *sternomastoid*: tell patient to push chin against your hand (away from the side of the lump) eg *trapezius*: tell patient to shrug his/her shoulders as you push down	*?fixation to underlying muscle* *?situated deep to muscle*
Examine for cervical lymphadenopathy (as above)	*?associated lymphadenopathy*

D. Examination of a salivary gland

ACTION	NOTE
Assess as for any lump (pages 26–28)	*?position* *?shape* *?colour* *?size* *?temperature* *?surface* *?edge* *?consistency*
Look inside the mouth: observe submandibular papillae (on either side of the frenulum) and the parotid duct orifice (opposite the crown of the second upper molar tooth)	Duct orifice: *?inflamed* *?pus/exudate*
Feel inside the mouth: bimanually palpate submandibular gland	A box of plastic gloves nearby suggests this is expected *?relation to tongue* *?relation to floor of mouth* *?tenderness*
Feel along duct	*?stone*
If you suspect enlargement of the parotid gland, test 7th nerve: 'screw up your eyes; blow out your cheeks; whistle'	*?facial nerve palsy*

TYPICAL CASES

1. MIDLINE NECK SWELLINGS

You should memorise a list of midline neck swellings:

COMMON	• Thyroid swellings • Thyroglossal cyst
UNCOMMON	• Lymph nodes • Sublingual dermoid cyst • Plunging ranula • Pharyngeal pouch • Subhyoid bursa • Carcinoma of larynx/trachea/oesophagus

Case I: Goitre

Revise the causes of a goitre:

a. **Physiological**

- Puberty
- Pregnancy

b. **Simple colloid goitre and multinodular goitre**
Note: these have the same underlying pathogenesis and a *multifactorial aetiology*:

- Goitregens
- Dyshormogenesis
- Iodine deficiency (epidemic, endemic)
- Autoimmune

c. **Autoimmune thyroid disease**

- Hashimoto's thyroiditis
- Graves' disease

d. **Other thyroiditides**

- de Quervain's (acute)
- Riedel's (chronic fibrosing)

e. Tumours

(i) Benign
(ii) Malignant: primary (carcinoma); secondary (lymphoma)

f. Other

- Tuberculosis
- Sarcoidosis

Note that if you feel a single nodule, you may be feeling the following:

- One nodule of a multinodular goitre
- An enlarged lobe (eg malignant infiltration; Hashimoto's thyroiditis)
- A true single nodule, ie a neoplasm. This may be *benign* (adenoma: functional or non-functional) or *malignant*.

You may be asked about the different kinds of primary thyroid cancers:

TYPE	NOTE
Papillary	Lump may be situated anterolaterally: otherwise known as 'lateral aberrant thyroid'; actually an involved lymph node
Follicular	Ask about bone pain (metastasises via blood)
Medullary	Lump feels stony hard due to amyloid infiltration
Anaplastic	Usually middle-aged or elderly patients Not a discrete lump because of infiltration into surrounding tissues
Malignant lymphoma	Associated with long standing Hashimoto's thyroiditis

Assess thyroid status independently: you are expected to know the common causes of hyper and hypothyroidism:

	CAUSE	NOTE
Hyperthyroidism	Graves' disease	• Autoimmune • Younger patients • Goitre is diffusely enlarged with bruit
	Multinodular goitre	• Older patients
	Functioning adenoma	• Rare • Most are non-functioning
Hypothyroidism	Primary myxoedema	• Autoimmune • Older patients • No goitre
	Hashimoto's thyroiditis	• Autoimmune • Younger patients • Rubbery goitre • At an early stage, patient may be hyperthyroid

Investigation: Determine levels of TSH T3 and T4 (euthyroid: normal TSH; hyperthyroid: TSH↓ T3↑; hypothyroid TSH↑ T4↓), thyroid antibodies for thyroiditis, ultrasound to differentiate cystic and nodular disease, CT and MRI to identify infiltration, fine needle aspiration and histological examination.

Treatment: Iodine for deficiency; remove goitrogens; suppress TSH with Thryoxine in multinodular goitres (can lead to 70% reduction in size). Surgery for retrosternal extension, tracheal compression and malignant tumours. Antithyroid treatment for hyperthyroidism, (usually long-term carbimazole with the addition of propranolol in severe cases). Surgery for relapse, if age <40 years; radioiodine in older patients, add two-week course of Lugol's iodine to drug management pre-operatively. Pregnancy: change antithyroid treatment to thiouracil; surgery safest in second trimester.

Case 2: Thyroglossal cyst

This is a spherical midline lump. It feels hard and the edge is clearly defined. Ask the patient to stick out his/her tongue: the lump will move *up* due to its attachment to the fibrous remnants of the thyroglossal tract.

Note its position: is it suprahyoid or infrahyoid?

You may find it difficult to fluctuate and to transilluminate.

Clinical diagnosis aided by imaging, particularly the need to define glossal extension.

Investigation: The clinical diagnosis is aided by imaging which is particularly important in defining glossal extension.

Treatment: Excision of cyst and whole tract. This may loop behind the hyoid bone requiring resection of the body, and following the tract into the base of the tongue.

2. LATERAL NECK SWELLINGS

Don't forget that an asymmetrical thyroid swelling may *appear* as a lateral neck swelling.

Otherwise, think of a lateral swelling as derived from paired lateral structures. Don't forget that lymph nodes are by far the most common cause.

	ANTERIOR TRIANGLE	POSTERIOR TRIANGLE
Lymph nodes	• Lymph node • Cold abscess*	• Lymph node • Cold abscess*
Salivary glands	• Submandibular swelling • Parotid swelling	
Cystic structures	Branchial cyst	Cystic hygroma
Vascular structures	• Carotid body tumour • Carotid artery aneurysm	Subclavian artery aneurysm
Other structures	Sternomastoid 'tumour' (ischaemic contracture)	Tumour of clavicle

* Note: a cold abscess arises from TB involvement of the nodes: the caseating nodes *point*, weakening the overlying tissue and then *burst*, causing a 'collar-stud' abscess.

Case 3: Cervical lymphadenopathy

You are likely to be asked the differential diagnosis:

	LOCALISED LYMPHADENOPATHY	GENERALISED LYMPHADENOPATHY
Infective	• Tonsillitis • Laryngitis • Infected skin lesion, eg sebaceous cyst • TB • Toxoplasmosis	(i) Acute • Infectious mononucleosis • Cytomegalovirus (ii) Chronic • TB • Brucellosis • Secondary syphilis • HIV
Neoplastic	Metastases from carcinoma of: • Head and neck • Breast • Chest • Abdomen	(i) Lymphoma • Hodgkin's • Non-Hodgkin's (ii) Leukaemias eg CLL
Other		• Amyloidosis • Sarcoidosis

Treatment: Identify the aetiology by clinical diagnosis which may be aided by fine needle aspiration, or excision biopsy; search for primary site.

Case 4: Salivary gland swelling

You may be given a patient with enlargement of the parotid or submandibular glands.
 Be able to classify the causes of salivary gland enlargement:

a. Infection: (sialoadenitis)
 (i) *Acute*
 - Viral
 - Bacterial
 (ii) *Recurrent*
 - Obstructive: calculus, stricture
 - Non-obstructive: children, menopausal females
 (iii) *Chronic*
 - Tuberculosis
 - Actinomycosis

b. Autoimmune
 - Sicca syndrome
 - Sjögren's syndrome

c. Calculi (sialolithiasis)

d. Cysts
 - Simple cysts (parotid)
 - Mucous retention cysts

e. Infiltration
 - Sarcoidosis

f. Systemic disease
 - Alcoholic liver cirrhosis
 - Diabetes mellitus
 - Pancreatitis
 - Acromegaly
 - Malnutrition

g. Drugs
 - Phenothiazines
 - Phenylbutazone

h. Allergy
 - Iodine

i. Malignancy
- Benign
- Intermediate
- Malignant

Remember.
- 80% of salivary *neoplastic* conditions occur in the parotid gland.
- Most *stones* occur in the *submandibular* gland.

The most likely cause of parotid enlargement is a benign mixed parotid tumour. Occasionally you will see a Warthin's tumour. The following characteristics distinguish these two tumours:

	MIXED PAROTID TUMOUR (PLEOMORPHIC ADENOMA)	WARTHIN'S TUMOUR
Position	Just above and anterior to the angle of the jaw	Slightly lower: lower border of mandible
Consistency	Rubbery-hard	Soft
Mobility	+	++
Fluctuant?	No	Yes

You may be asked how you would clinically assess the *malignancy* of a parotid tumour. The distinguishing features are:

- Short presentation
- Painful
- Hyperaemic and hot skin
- Hard consistency
- Fixed to skin and underlying muscle
- Irregular surface and indistinct edge
- Invasion of facial nerve

Treatment: Treat infection with appropriate antibiotic. Dilate strictures, remove stones and marsupialise orifice. Watch small benign tumours. In surgery, protect facial nerve by excising local superficial lump with or without a surrounding cuff of normal tissue. Remove tumour or superficial parotidectomy. Total parotidectomy, sacrifice nerve for infiltrating lesions, neck dissection for involved nodes +/- adjunctive radiotherapy.

Case 5: Cervical rib

This rarely comes up in examinations.

The lump is only occasionally palpable, just above the clavicle. It may be pulsatile due to the elevated and sometimes dilated subclavian artery.

Look out for neurological and vascular features:

a. **Neurological features** (more common)
   ● Pain in C8 and T1 dermatomes
   ● Wasting and weakness of small muscles of the hand

b. **Vascular features** (rarer)
   ● Raynaud's phenomenon
   ● Rest pain
   ● Trophic changes
   ● Gangrene

Treatment: Excise symptomatic ribs. Associated vascular lesions may require local resection of aneurysm, distal thrombectomy and sympathectomy.

Case 6: Carotid body tumour

This is a rare condition but may come up in the examination as a short case. The tumour feels hard and is otherwise known as a 'potato tumour'. The position is shown opposite.

You may feel pulsation. This may result from the following sources:

   ● Internal carotid artery (transmitted)
   ● External carotid artery (running superficially)
   ● Tumour itself (intrinsic vascularity)

Ask about blackouts, transient paralysis and paraesthesia.

Check the other side: the tumour is often bilateral.

Treatment: Observe small, often bilateral tumours. Excise enlarging, symptomatic and invasive tumours. May need replacement of carotid artery. Essential to make the diagnosis pre-operatively, so that a vascular surgeon is involved.

Case 7. Branchial cyst/sinus/fistula

Note that, although these are *developmental*, arising from remnants of the second pharyngeal pouch, they present in young adults.

The cyst has a distinct edge and a smooth surface. Depending on its contents, it may or may not transilluminate.

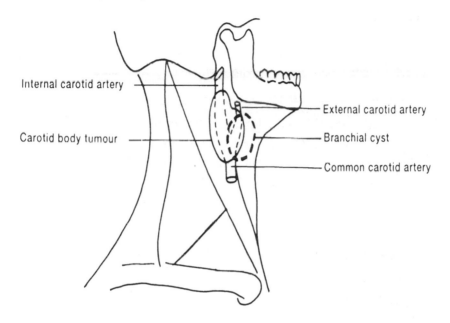

You may be shown a branchial sinus or fistula – a small dimple in the skin, at the junction of the middle and lower third of the anterior edge of sternomastoid.

- Ask the patient to swallow: this will make it more obvious.
- Ask about discharge.

Know the *definitions* of a sinus and a fistula:

a. Sinus: a blindly ending track, leading away from an epithelial surface into surrounding tissue, lined by epithelial or granulation tissue.
(In this instance, there is no closing off of the second branchial cleft, although the upper end is obliterated.)

b. Fistula: an abnormal tract connecting two epithelial surfaces, lined by epithelial or granulation tissue.
(In this instance, the fistula connects skin to the oropharynx, just behind the tonsil.)

Treatment: Complete excision.

POPULAR VIVA QUESTIONS

1. What are the causes of cervical lymphadenopathy?

2. What are the possible causes of a lump in the anterior triangle of the neck?

3. What are the causes of a thyroid swelling?

4. What are the causes of hyper and hypothyroidism?

5. What are the indications for the surgical management of hyperthyroidism?

6. What precautions would you take in preparing a patient with hyperthyroidism for surgery?

7. What are the complications of thyroidectomy?

8. What kinds of thyroid malignancy do you know?

9. What are the sites of the openings of the submandibular and parotid ducts into the mouth?

10. What are the causes of stones in the salivary ducts? Where are they most likely to form?

11. What is the most common tumour of the parotid gland? How should it be managed?

12. What clinical features distinguish a benign from a malignant salivary tumour?

13. What are the complications of surgery to the parotid gland?

Answers on pages 173–175

8: The breast

Your patient in either the long or short case may be a woman complaining of pain or a lump in her breast.

THE HISTORY

Bring out the following points when presenting under 'history of presenting complaint':

Breast lump

- When did you notice the lump? How did you notice it?
- Has the lump *changed* since you first noticed it? How?
- Is it painful?
- Have you had any breast lumps in the past?
- Has anyone in your family had breast lumps?

Nipple discharge

- Do you have discharge from *both* nipples?
- What colour is the discharge?
- Have you breast-fed recently?

Hormonal factors

- Does the lump change with your menstrual cycle or at different times in the month?
- When did you start your periods? (*menarche*)
  If relevant, When did you stop your periods? (*menopause*)
- How many children do you have? Did you breast-feed them? Were there any problems?
- Have you ever been on the pill or hormone replacement therapy?

THE EXAMINATION

The usual instruction given in the short case is to 'examine the breasts'. Proceed as below.

Occasionally, you may be asked just to feel and describe a lump in the breast, in which case you should proceed as described on pages 26–28. Remember at all times to be sensitive and to avoid discomfort and embarrassment. Cover the breasts up when you are examining other systems.

'Examine this patient's breasts'

ACTION	NOTE
Introduce yourself	
Ask permission to examine the patient	
Expose the breasts with the patient at 45° to the horizontal	
LOOK	
Stand opposite the patient	
Ask her to raise her arms slowly above her head	*?asymmetry* *?nipple retraction* *?skin puckering*
FEEL	If your patient has pendulous breasts, lie her flatter. Rest the arm of the breast to be examined behind her head. Ask her to lean slightly to the other side
Ask the patient to point to the lump with one finger	
Ask if the breasts are tender	

Start with the normal breast
Palpate *systematically*, each
quadrant in turn and then centrally
around the nipple
Palpate with the flat of your fingers

Palpate the *affected* breast:
all quadrants except that of the
lump itself

Try to elicit any discharge
by gently squeezing the nipple

site: *?nipple segment*
colour: *?red*
        ?green
        ?yellow
        ?clear

ASSESS THE LUMP

Omit this section if no lump is
found on examination

Feel and measure the lump

overlying skin: *?warm*

texture: *?stony-hard*
          ?rubbery-hard
          ?soft

shape/size: *?exact dimensions*

Try to move the skin
overlying the lump

skin: *?no movement* (implies
     fixation)

     *?wrinkles at extremes of
     movement* (implies tethering)

Ask your patient to rest her hand
lightly on the hip of the same side.
Move the lump with your finger
and thumb:
- up and down
- at right angles

?mobility

Ask her to press hard on her hip
Move the lump as above

movement of lump: *?reduced on
contraction of pectorales muscles*
(indicates attachment to muscle)

Examine the axillae:
hold the patient's right elbow in
your right hand
Take the weight of her forearm

Palpate the walls:
- medial
- anterior
- lateral
- posterior
- apical

If in doubt, palpate from behind
patient

?associated lymphadenopathy

Repeat on the other side

Palpate the cervical nodes

Palpate the supraclavicular fossae
and behind sternomastoid

ASSESS FURTHER

Palpate the liver

?hepatomegaly
?knobbly edge

Percuss down the back
Ask if it is tender at any point

?tenderness, suggestive of bone
metastases

Percuss the lung bases

?dull

COMPLETE THE EXAMINATION

Cover the patient's breasts with
a sheet

Turn to the examiner and present
your findings

TYPICAL CASES

Breast lumps come up as long (OSLER) and short (OSCE) cases. Revise the causes of a breast lump:

CAUSE	EXAMPLE	
Physiological	Fibroadenosis	
Neoplastic	(i) Benign	• Fibroadenoma • Duct papilloma • Phylloides tumour
	(ii) Malignant	• Primary carcinoma • Secondary carcinoma
Traumatic	Fat necrosis	
Infective	Cellulitis Abscesses	

You should be able to differentiate clinically between the commoner lumps:

	CARCINOMA	FIBROADENOMA	FIBROADENOSIS
No. of Lumps	1	1+	1+
Pain	Rare	Rare	Common: varies with menstrual cycle
Irregularity	++	−	−
Hardness	+++	++	+

Case 1: Breast carcinoma

This is a very common case. Remember the classical features:

a. **Age 35+**

b. **Positive family history**

c. **Lump:**
- Stony hard
- Irregular edge
- Tethered/fixed to skin* (see table on page 64)
- Immobile

d. Nipple:
- Inverted
- Distorted
- Peu d'orange
- Bloody discharge
- Red, encrusted, oozing (Paget's disease)

e. Lymphadenopathy

f. Features of metastases:
- Backache
- Breathlessness
- Jaundice
- Malaise and weight loss

* Note: the differences between tethering and fixation:

	TETHERING	FIXATION
Infiltration	Along ligaments of Astley Cooper	To skin
Mobility	Some	None
Skin	Dimples at extremes of movement	Cannot be moved over lump
Prognosis	Better	Worse

Remember that the signs of breast carcinoma may be mimicked by other conditions. Consider the following:

a. Hard irregular lumps: fat necrosis and chronic mastitis.

b. Nipple inversion: this may be long-standing or congenital.

c. Nipple discharge: see Case 4.

d. Nipple skin changes: differentiate Paget's disease from eczema:

	PAGET'S DISEASE	ECZEMA
Cause	Spread of intraductal carcinoma to epidermis	Atopy
Bilateral?	No	Yes
Itchy?	No	Yes
Vesicular?	No	Yes

Treatment: Staging of breast cancer is valuable in both choice of treatment and as a prognostic indicator. Stages 1 to 4 have a TNM classification superimposed.

Stage 1: early disease confined to the breast ($T_1 < 2$ cm);

Stage 2: axillary nodal spread (T_2 2–5 cm N_1); stages 1 and 2 are classified as early disease.

Stage 3a: locally advanced disease

Stage 3b: chest wall involvement ($T_3 > 5$ cm, T_4 skin and chest wall involvement N_2 fixed nodes N_3 ipsilateral internal mammary nodes)

Stage 4: extension of disease beyond the breast (M_1).

Treatment of early disease is wide local excision with radiotherapy, or simple mastectomy with nodal sampling or clearance below the axillary vein and medial to pectoralis minor muscle. Treatment of advanced disease is by radiotherapy and endocrinal chemotherapy directed at symptomatic site or used to downstage locally advanced disease prior to surgery.

The Nottingham Prognostic Index (NPI) uses: histological types and grades, hormonal receptor status and the presence of oncogenes (detected by epidermal growth factor receptor and a cerb B2 receptor). A score of less than three with this system suggests a greater than 85% ten year survival. This falls to less than 20% for scores greater than five.

Case 2: Fibroadenoma

A woman with a fibroadenoma will usually be young (peak 25–35 years).

There may be more than one lump. The lumps are small and rubbery-hard. They are very mobile and are therefore also known as 'breast mice'.

Investigation: includes ultrasound and fine needle cytology.

Treatment: Age <35: stop hormonal contraceptives and reassure. Age >35: excision biopsy.

Case 3: Fibroadenosis

This condition is very common and borders on physiological change.

It occurs in women of reproductive age, peak 35–45 years. Ask specifically about variation with the menstrual cycle.

There are many presentations:

- Single lump (solid or cystic)
- Multiple lumps or generalised nodularity
- Cyclical breast pain
- Nipple discharge (clear, white or green)

Treatment: Age <35: ultrasound. Age >40: mammography to exclude neoplasia. Stop hormonal contraceptives or HRT. A trial of Evening Primrose capsules. Where cysts have been aspirated, core needle biopsy or excision biopsy is used to assess any residual lesion.

Case 4: Nipple discharge

Ask yourself the following key questions:

a. Is the discharge true?
Eczema, Paget's disease and fistulae all cause discharges which do not arise from the ducts themselves.

b. Is the discharge significant?
For a discharge to be significant, it must have occurred:
- spontaneously
- over a year after stopping breast-feeding
- more than once

c. Is the discharge worrying?
The following features suggest carcinoma:
- *Unilateral* discharge
- *Bloody* discharge
- Discharge arising from a *single* duct (single nipple segment)

The colour of the discharge may give you a clue as to the cause:

COLOUR	NATURE	CAUSE
Red	Blood	• Ductal carcinoma • Duct papilloma
Green	Cell debris	• Fibroadenosis • Duct ectasia
Yellow	Exudate	• Fibroadenosis • Abscess
White	Milk	• Lactation

Investigation: Includes cytology of the discharge and triple assessment (palpation, breast imaging and fine needle cytology of any underlying lesion). This is followed by core needle biopsy of any area of equivocal findings.

Treatment: Malignancy is managed as outlined in Case 1 or enrolment onto a screening programme.

Based on these results of investigation.

POPULAR VIVA QUESTIONS

1. What is a fibroadenoma?

2. How may fibroadenosis present?

3. What benign breast diseases come into the differential diagnosis of breast cancer?

4. What are the advantages of mammography for breast cancer screening?

5. What are the presenting features of breast carcinoma?

6. Where does breast cancer spread?

7. What is Paget's disease of the nipple?

8. What are the causes of nipple discharge?

9. What do you understand by the term 'early breast cancer'?

10. How would you manage a woman with early breast cancer?

11. What are the advantages of lumpectomy over mastectomy for breast cancer?

12. What is advanced breast cancer?

13. What are the alternative treatments in advanced breast cancer?

Answers on pages 175–176

9: The gastrointestinal tract

THE HISTORY

Give a succinct and chronological report of your patient's presenting complaint. Bring out the following aspects in your presentation:

The history of the patient's pain

(see page 25)

The history of the patient's lump/swelling

(see page 25)

Remainder of systemic enquiry of the GIT

Ask about the following symptoms:
- Dysphagia
- Dyspepsia
- Abdominal swelling/distension
- Nausea and vomiting
- Appetite and weight loss
- Change in bowel habit

Remember that diarrhoea/constipation are not precise words: ask what is normal for your patient.
Report on the stool:
?consistency
?frequency
?colour
?blood (?mixed in ?on the surface ?on the toilet paper)
?anal discharge/pruritus ani

THE EXAMINATION

Listen carefully to the instruction. In a short case, you may be asked to 'examine the gastrointestinal system' or 'examine the abdomen'.

As with the examination of any system, always start with the hands. You may be stopped at this stage and asked to proceed to the abdomen itself. Occasionally, you may be instructed to 'palpate the abdomen', in which case beginning with the hands will only antagonise the examiners.

Note the following points:

- Make sure your hands are warm

- Don't hurt your patient: during palpation, keep looking at his/her face for wincing

- Don't forget the following points on account of exam nerves:

  - Percussion of the upper border of the liver (*normally 5th intercostal space. May be displaced downwards with hyperexpansion of the chest*)
  - Groin
  - External genitalia
  - Statement that you would normally perform a rectal examination

Also remember the **3 A**s:

a. Aortic aneurysm
b. Ascites
c. Auscultation

'Examine this patient's gastrointestinal system'

ACTION	NOTE
Introduce yourself	
Ask permission to examine the patient	
Expose the abdomen with the patient lying flat with one pillow supporting the head	Include the inguinal regions but not the genitalia

1. Preliminary assessment

ACTION	NOTE

Look at both hands	nails: *?clubbing ?leuconychia*
	palms: *?palmar erythema*
	           ?Dupuytren's contracture
	           ?pallor of skin creases

Ask patient to stretch out arms with the wrists cocked up	*?liver flap*
Look at the eyes	sclera: *?jaundice* conjunctiva: *?pallor*
Look at the mouth	*?telangiectasia* (indicates hereditary haemorrhagic telangiectasia) *?perioral pigmentation* (indicates Peutz-Jegher's syndrome)
Look at the angles of the mouth	*?angular stomatitisation* (can occur in young, but sign of iron deficiency and debilitation in the aged)
Ask patient to stick out tongue	*?dehydration* *?coated tongue*
Smell breath	*?ketosis* *?halitosis*
Palpate cervical lymph nodes	In this case, it is not necessary to examine from behind the patient *?cervical lymphadenopathy*
Show the examiner you are paying particular attention to the *left* supraclavicular fossa	*?Virchow's node/Troisier's sign*
Look at the chest	skin: *?spider naevi* *?purpura*
Palpate gently around the nipples	*?gynaecomastia*

2. The abdomen

<u>ACTION</u> | <u>NOTE</u>

LOOK

Stand at the end of the bed

skin: *?scars*
       ?stoma site
       ?visible veins
shape: *?distended*
       ?scaphoid
       ?visible peristalsis
       ?visible masses

Ask patient to take a deep breath, draw in the abdomen and cough

?pain (limiting movement)
?asymmetry (mass, discomfort)
?mass (made more obvious)

FEEL

Palpate with your palm and the flat of your fingers
Keep your forearm level with the abdominal wall

You may need to kneel down if the bed is low

a. Preliminary palpation

Ask if the abdomen is tender

Palpate each quadrant lightly

?tenderness
?guarding
?rigidity

Palpate each quadrant more deeply, leaving the tender areas until last

?deep tenderness
?masses
?palpable viscera

b. Assessment of a mass

If you find a mass, determine its characteristics at this stage (pages 26–28)	?*size* ?*shape* ?*surface* ?*edge* ?*consistency* ?*percussion note* ?*bruit/bowel sounds*

c. Assessment of organomegaly

(i) *Liver*

Palpate the liver, beginning in the right iliac fossa As patient breathes in and out, move your hand upwards in stages until you reach the costal margin	?*hepatomegaly* ?*smooth edge* ?*knobbly edge* ?*consistency* ?*tenderness* ?*pulsatility*
Percuss out the liver: lower and upper borders	?*dull*

(ii) *Spleen*

Palpate the spleen, beginning in the right iliac fossa As patient breathes in and out, move your hand towards the tip of the tenth rib	?*splenomegaly*
On reaching the costal margin, place your left hand around the lower left rib cage Palpate with your right hand in the midaxillary line	If you still cannot feel the spleen, ask the patient to roll towards you
Percuss for an enlarged spleen	?*dull*

(iii) *Kidneys*

Palpate each kidney: position one hand behind patient's loin and the other hand just above ASIS	Your hand should be *well* behind patient's loin
Ask patient to breath deeply	?*enlarged kidneys*

(iv) *Aortic aneurysm*
Place two hands along the midline, just above the umbilicus

?expansile pulsation
?can you get above it
(if so infra-renal probably is anyway)
?transverse diameter

d. Examination of groin and external genitalia

Place your fingers over the inguinal and femoral orifices
Ask patient to cough

?cough impulse

Feel inguinal lymph nodes

?inguinal lymphadenopathy

Feel testes

?atrophy
?mass

e. Examination for ascites

This is only necessary if the abdomen is distended

(i) *Shifting dullness*
Percuss over the abdomen
Start centrally and move to the flanks

Keep your finger in the sagittal plane

Locate the point on one side where the percussion note changes from resonant to dull

Ask patient to roll over on that side, keeping your hand in this position

Percuss again

?has area of dullness moved

(ii) *Fluid thrill*
Ask patient to place the edge of his/her hand along the midline

Flick one side while feeling the other side

?thrill

LISTEN

Auscultate abdomen over at least three different areas	*?bowel sounds* *?pitch* *?increased/decreased*
Listen along the course of the aorta and iliac arteries and in the renal areas	*?bruits*

SAY

'I would like to: • do a rectal examination • examine the urine with a dipstick'	*?mass* *?proteinuria* *?haematuria* *?glucose*

COMPLETE THE EXAMINATION

Cover the patient up

Turn to the examiner

Present your findings

TYPICAL CASES

You are unlikely to meet a patient with an 'acute abdomen' in either the short or long case. However, you should revise the causes of acute abdominal pain for discussion in the clinical examination and viva.

In the long case, you may meet patients with abdominal symptoms but few signs. Examples are patients with peptic ulcers, chronic cholecystitis (and bouts of biliary colic), chronic pancreatitis, diverticular disease, irritable bowel syndrome and inflammatory bowel disease.

You may also have a patient with jaundice. In a surgical examination, the most likely cause will be post-hepatic 'obstructive' jaundice. However, when asked the differential diagnosis, mention pre-hepatic and hepatocellular causes.

The main physical signs, to be picked up in both the long and short case, are scars and stomas, organomegaly, masses and distension. This section revises the differential diagnosis of these signs.

1. SCARS AND STOMAS

Scars

Always look very carefully for abdominal scars: old ones are surprisingly easy to miss, especially in hirsute men. It is particularly easy to miss a Pfannenstiel incision, appendicectomy scar and a left nephrectomy scar (look well over the left loin).

You should know the usual sites:

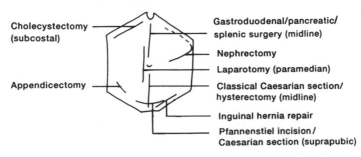

Cholecystectomy (subcostal)

Gastroduodenal/pancreatic/ splenic surgery (midline)

Nephrectomy

Laparotomy (paramedian)

Appendicectomy

Classical Caesarian section/ hysterectomy (midline)

Inguinal hernia repair

Pfannenstiel incision/ Caesarian section (suprapubic)

Short (1–1.5 cm) scars along the midline and elsewhere may indicate laparoscopic procedures.

Stomas

You should understand the differences between ileostomies and colostomies:

	ILEOSTOMY	COLOSTOMY
Type	Permanent only	Temporary or permanent
Indications	• Ulcerative colitis • Crohn's disease • Inherited polyposis coli	• Colorectal carcinoma • Diverticular disease
Appearance	Spout of mucosa	Mucosa sutured to skin
Position	Right iliac fossa	• Permanent: left iliac fossa • Temporary: right hypochondrium or left iliac fossa
Effluent	Continuous	Intermittent
Complications	• Fluid and electrolyte imbalance	• Ischaemia • Obstruction • Skin erosion • Recurrent disease at stoma site • Bowel prolapse • Parastomal hernia

2. ORGANOMEGALY

Case 1: Hepatomegaly

In a surgical examination, the most common cause of hepatomegaly is metastases. The patient may or may not be jaundiced. Your examiner will expect you to know the other causes of hepatomegaly.

Common causes in the United Kingdom include the following:

- Metastases
- Congestive cardiac failure (right-sided)
- Cirrhosis (not in later stages, when liver shrinks and is impalpable)
- Infections, eg viral hepatitis, infectious mononucleosis

Go through your surgical sieve (page 16) to retrieve rarer causes.

Your *description* of the liver should help in your differential diagnosis:

a. **Edge:** (i) *Smooth*
- Cirrhosis
- Congestive heart failure

(ii) *Knobbly*
- Secondary carcinoma
- Macronodular cirrhosis (rare)

b. **Consistency:** *Hard* if metastases

c. **Tenderness:** Occurs when capsule is distended:
- Congestive heart failure
- Hepatitis
- Hepatocellular carcinoma
- AV malformation
- Alcoholic hepatitis (rare)

d. **Pulsatility:**
- Tricuspid regurgitation

See Treatment following Case 3.

Case 2: Splenomegaly

If your patient has splenomegaly, you may well be asked to justify your diagnosis in terms of its five distinguishing characteristics:

- Descends towards the right iliac fossa
- Moves down on inspiration
- Palpable anterior notch
- Cannot get above it
- Dull to percussion (continuous with area of splenic dullness over 9th, 10th and 11th ribs, behind posterior axillary line)

Have a list of causes of massive, moderate and mild splenomegaly. As always, give the common causes in the UK first (eg myelofibrosis rather than kala-azar, for massive splenomegaly).

MASSIVE	MODERATE	MILD
	As for massive *plus*	As for moderate *plus*
• Myelofibrosis	• Haemolytic anaemia	• Infectious mononucleosis
• Chronic granulocytic leukaemia	• Chronic lymphocytic leukaemia	• Myeloproliferative disorders
• Malaria	• Lymphomas	• Pernicious anaemia
• Kala-azar	• Portal hypertension	• Amyloidosis
		• Sarcoidosis
		• Rheumatoid arthritis (Felty's syndrome)

Although many of these causes of splenomegaly are 'medical', your patient may be awaiting a splenectomy because of its complications: *hypersplenism* leads to both pooling and destruction by the reticulo-endothelial system of haemopoietic cells, causing a pancytopaenia. Be aware of the potential problems of splenectomy, eg infection with capsulated bacteria such as pneumococcus. Know about the measures to reduce such complications (Pneumovax immunisation, prophylactic penicillin).

See Treatment following Case 3.

Case 3: Hepatosplenomegaly

Causes of enlargement of the spleen as well as the liver include some of the above, eg lymphoma, leukaemias, infections, amyloidosis and sarcoidosis. The most likely case in an examination is cirrhosis with associated portal hypertension.

Treatment for cases 1, 2 and 3: Management of most of the listed diseases is that of the underlying cause. Surgery of hepatomegaly may include drainage of abscesses, segmental resection of tumours and occasionally transplantation. Indications for splenectomy include septicaemic abscesses, schistosomiasis, tropical splenomegaly, hydatid cysts, Gaucher's disease, myelofibrosis, thalassaemia, sickle cell disease, lymphoma, embolic infarction, splenic artery or venous thrombosis, and possibly hereditary spherocytosis, idiopathic splenomegaly, thrombocytopaenic purpura and solitary or polycystic disease.

Case 4: Enlarged kidneys

Remember that in slim people, the lower pole of the right kidney may be palpable.

Know the characteristics of a renal swelling:

- Ballotable (*bimanually palpable*)
- Descends vertically
- Moves down on respiration
- Resonant to percussion due to overlying colon (*not always*: some parts may be dull)
- Can get above it (*rarely*)

Another popular question is to differentiate between an enlarged left kidney and a palpable spleen:

	KIDNEY	SPLEEN
Descent on inspiration?	Vertically	Towards right iliac fossa
Ballotable?	Yes	No
Notch present?	No	Yes
Can you ever get above it?	Occasionally	No
Percussion note?	Resonant (usually)	Dull

In finals, the most common cause of *bilateral* renal enlargement is polycystic kidneys. These may be extremely large and feel lobulated because of the multiple cysts. If you suspect this condition:

- Ask about family history (inheritance is *autosomal dominant*)
- Take the blood pressure
- Ask to examine the urine (?*haematuria* ?*proteinuria* ?*casts*) – try to palpate a liver which may also be polycystic
- Look for a third nerve palsy due to pressure from an associated posterior communicating artery Berry aneurysm

Other causes of bilateral renal enlargement are bilateral hydronephrosis and amyloidosis.

Causes of *unilateral* renal enlargement include the following:

- Hydronephrosis
- Simple benign cysts
- Hypertrophy
- Tumour, eg renal cell carcinoma

A transplanted kidney will usually be found in an iliac fossa.

Treatment: Progressive renal failure from polycystic disease may require transplantation; hydronephrosis: drainage and treatment of the cause; renal cell carcinoma: nephrectomy with removal of intravenous extension and possibly pulmonary metastases.

3. MASSES

Revise pages 26–28 for the description of any mass.

As many masses are visible on careful observation of the abdomen, do not forget to look first.

List and revise the causes of masses in each segment of the abdomen.

Case 5: Mass in right hypochondrium

The causes of a mass in the right hypochondrium include the following:

- Hepatomegaly
- Enlarged gallbladder
- Enlarged right kidney
- Colonic mass

Revise the causes of an enlarged gallbladder:

a. **Obstruction of cystic duct**: mucocoele or empyema.

b. **Obstruction of the common bile duct**, eg cancer of the head of the pancreas.

Remember *Courvoisier's law*:

'If the gallbladder is palpable and the patient is jaundiced, the obstruction of the bile duct causing the jaundice is unlikely to be due to a stone.'

c. **Gallbladder mass**: inflammation with surrounding adherent omentum.

Also note the characteristics of an enlarged gallbladder:

- Appears from the tip of the 9th rib
- Cannot get between it and the liver edge
- Dull to percussion
- Smooth surface
- Moves down on inspiration (not always true of gallbladder mass)

See Treatment following Case 10.

Case 6: Mass in epigastrium

The two most important causes are carcinoma of the stomach and pancreatic masses (pseudocyst, carcinoma). An aortic aneurysm is situated deep to the umbilicus, but may also fill the epigastrium.

Two 'catches' are:

a. **Liver:** either left lobe or a post-necrotic nodule of a cirrhotic liver.

b. **Large recti:** these appear to enlarge when the patient sits forwards.

You should suspect gastric or pancreatic carcinoma in a cachectic patient complaining of pain, dyspepsia, anorexia and significant weight loss. You may not always feel a mass.

Note the characteristics of a *gastric* carcinoma:

- Hard, irregular
- Cannot get above it
- Moves with respiration

Think immediately of checking for a left supraclavicular node (*Virchow's node/Troisier's sign*).

Gastric carcinoma may be difficult to differentiate from a pancreatic pseudocyst which, although uncommon, crops up disproportionately in examinations. The characteristics of a pancreatic pseudocyst are as follows:

- Cannot get above it
- Indistinct lower border
- Resonant to percussion
- Moves slightly with respiration

See Treatment following Case 10.

Case 7: Mass in left hypochondrium

The most common cause is an enlarged spleen. Other causes are a pancreatic mass (carcinoma of tail) and an enlarged left kidney.

See Treatment following Case 10.

Case 8: **Right loin**	Case 9: **Umbilical region**	Case 10: **Left loin**
• Enlarged right kidney • Enlarged liver • Enlarged gall bladder See Treatment following Case 10	• Small bowel mass (nodal or omental) • Cancer of transverse colon • Aortic aneurysm See Treatment following Case 10	• Enlarged left kidney • Enlarged spleen

Investigation for cases 5–10: Confirmation of the diagnosis in these areas can usually be obtained by imaging techniques. CT and MRI provide reliable diagnostic information on the liver, spleen, pancreas, kidneys and retroperitoneal structures, identifying inflammatory change as well as benign and malignant tumours, with or without invasion and secondary spread.

Treatment for cases 5–10: Aortic aneurysm: an abdominal aortic aneurysm is usually a clinical diagnosis; intervention by stenting or open surgery is considered in lesions of over 6 cm in diameter. Gall bladder: cholelithiasis is managed by cholecystectomy and exploration and evacuation of the common bile and hepatic ducts, possibly through endoscopic means. Pancreas: acute pancreatitis occasionally requires surgical débridement and drainage; malignant tumours of the body and tail of the pancreas are usually inoperable by the time of diagnosis; a lesion causing jaundice may still be resectable by a Whipple's procedure.

Case 11: Mass in right iliac fossa

A mass in the right iliac fossa is a common clinical case.

The most common causes are carcinoma of the caecum and Crohn's disease.

a. Carcinoma of caecum

Suspect this condition in an elderly patient who appears clinically anaemic. The mass is often well-defined and hard. It may be mobile or fixed. It is not usually tender.

b. Crohn's disease

This is usually seen in younger patients. The mass feels rubbery and non-tender and may be fairly mobile.

These are the less common causes:

- Appendix mass
- Ileocaecal TB
- Iliac lymphadenopathy
- Ovarian cyst
- Pelvic (transplanted) kidney

See Treatment following Case 12.

Case 12: Mass in left iliac fossa

The common causes are a loaded sigmoid colon (may be normally palpable, but particularly with constipation or diverticular disease, it can usually be indented) and carcinoma of the colon. Rarer causes are Crohn's disease and iliac lymphadenopathy. Again, don't forget gynaecological causes (eg an ovarian mass) or transplanted kidney.

a. Diverticular disease

You are unlikely to be given a patient with a diverticular abscess. However, patients with diverticular disease often have a palpable, tender sigmoid colon.

b. Carcinoma of colon

The patient normally presents with a change in bowel habit. The mass is usually hard.

Feel for an enlarged liver and listen for high-pitched bowel sounds (in the presence of any obstruction).

Treatment for cases 11 and 12: Most iliac fossa masses are related to lesions of the colon. Appendix abscesses may require drainage. Those extending laterally are allowed to resolve, followed after a few months, by interval appendicectomy. Medial extensions may give rise to further gut symptoms and may require a difficult surgical resection in the acute phase.

Obstruction from inflammatory bowel disease, diverticular disease or colonic malignancy may require emergency surgery with temporary colostomy with subsequent resection with or without restoration of gut continuity. It may also be possible to undertake definitive surgery, at the time of the initial emergency procedure. Fulminating toxic megacolon in ulcerative colitis is a serious emergency that may respond to steroids. Emergency surgery is directed at retroperitoneal decompression to avoid peritoneal contamination before total proctocolectomy.

Crohn's disease may require drainage of abscesses and resection of fistulae. The aim is to preserve as much bowel as possible.

Case 13: Suprapubic mass

Suprapubic masses are easily missed.

The two characteristics of a pelvic swelling are:

- Cannot get below it
- May be palpated bimanually on vaginal or rectal examination

The most common cause is an enlarged bladder. This has the following characteristics:

- Dull to percussion
- Fluid thrill
- Direct pressure produces desire to micturate

In the female, do not forget obstetric and gynaecological causes: the most frequent pelvic mass in the female is the pregnant uterus. Also consider a large ovarian cyst and uterine fibroids.

Manual examination improves diagnosis of obstetric and gynaecological causes.

Treatment: An enlarged bladder usually requires decompression by transurethral or suprapubic catheterisation. Emergency surgery may be required for ectopic pregnancies and complications of ovarian cysts. As much ovarian tissue as possible is preserved in the pre-menstrual years, but ovarian cancer requires extensive clearance, as well as a chemotherapeutic approach. Uterine cancer, fibroids and other lesions may require hysterectomy with or without oophorectomy.

Case 14: Abdominal distension

Remember the 5 Fs:

a. **Fetus:** very unlikely in a surgical examination but always consider in a woman of reproductive age.

b. **Flatus:** the abdomen is hyper-resonant; you may see visible peristalsis.

c. **Faeces:** you are unlikely to be given a patient with acute obstruction. However, chronic constipation is a common surgical problem. Beware – your patient may be complaining of diarrhoea and in fact be constipated (spurious diarrhoea).

Faeces have the following characteristics:

- Lie in the distribution of the colon
- Often form multiple separate masses
- Can be indented with digital pressure

d. **Fat:** usually obvious; deposition is in the lower half of the abdomen.

e. **Fluid:** ascites can be detected by two tests: fluid thrill and shifting dullness. The latter is more reliable because a fluid thrill is detected in any abdominal fluid-filled cavity.

Treatment: According to diagnosis (see treatment of cases 11 and 12). Ascites requires diagnostic aspiration if the etiology is unknown.

POPULAR VIVA QUESTIONS

1. What are the causes of:
   - dysphagia
   - hepatomegaly
   - splenomegaly
   - hepatosplenomegaly
   - jaundice
   - change in bowel habit
   - diarrhoea
   - constipation
   - haematemesis
   - melaena
   - blood PR
   - intestinal obstruction: *?in children ?in adults*
   - pruritis ani

2. Differentiate between tenderness, rebound tenderness, guarding and rigidity.

3. What is the difference between peritonism and peritonitis?

4. How do gallstones present?

5. How does presentation of carcinoma of the head of the pancreas differ from that of the tail of the pancreas?

6. What is the difference between diverticulosis and diverticulitis?

7. What are the complications of diverticular disease?

8. What are the differences between Crohn's disease and ulcerative colitis?

9. What are the local and general complications of inflammatory bowel disease?

10. What is Dukes' staging for colorectal cancer?

11. How does the presentation of carcinoma of the right side of the bowel differ from that of the left?

12. What are the symptoms of intestinal obstruction?

13. What are the extra-abdominal causes of acute abdominal pain?

Answers on pages 177–182

10: The groin and scrotum

THE HISTORY

Hernias and groin lumps are very popular short and OSCE cases. After examining a hernia, you may be instructed to ask the patient some additional questions. Structure them as follows:

The lump itself

(see page 25)

Predisposing causes

- Do you have a chronic cough/asthma/bronchitis?
- Do you do much heavy lifting?
- Do you have to strain to pass a motion?
  (Note that this may occur both with constipation and diarrhoea)
- Do you have difficulty passing water?

Potential complications (strangulation and obstruction)

- Does the lump become tender or painful?
- Do you have any abdominal pain?
- Have you vomited recently?
- Have you noticed your abdomen swelling/your clothes getting tighter?
- Are you constipated?

THE EXAMINATION

In a short case, you may be asked specifically to 'examine this hernia' or 'this scrotal lump', in which case you should examine as for any lump (pages

26–28) plus perform the additional assessment outlined below. If you are asked to 'examine the groin', follow the whole examination scheme.

Note the following points:

- You may see an inguinal lump you are certain is a hernia. However, always examine the scrotum as well. There may be dual pathology.
- Always examine both sides: 20% of hernias are bilateral.
- Try to distinguish between a direct and an indirect inguinal hernia. Some say that this is unimportant as it does not affect the patient's management. However, you cannot be faulted for being too thorough.

'Examine this patient's groin'

ACTION	NOTE
Introduce yourself	
Ask permission to examine the patient	If there is an *obvious* inguinoscrotal swelling, do not stand the patient up. Otherwise, examine with the patient standing
Expose the groin and external genitalia	

1. Examination of the external genitalia

LOOK

Observe the anterior aspect of the scrotum	skin: *?colour* swelling: *?inguinal ?scrotal*
Observe the posterior aspect of the scrotum, pulling on posterior skin, **not** the testes	

FEEL

Roll the testes *gently* between your thumb (in front) and index finger (behind)	*?both testes palpable*
Locate the epididymis (above and posterior to testis)	*?epididymal swelling*
Feel along the spermatic cord	*?cord swelling*

ASSESSMENT OF SWELLING

Define its characteristics (see pages 26–28)	*?size* *?shape* *?surface* *?consistency* *?fluctuant* *?transilluminable*
Try to locate its upper edge	*?can you get above it*
Try to feel testis	*?testis separate from swelling*

2. Examination for hernias

ACTION	NOTE
Stand to one side of the patient who should be standing (see above) Locate the pubic tubercle Place one hand behind patient and the examining hand over the swelling	If no swelling is seen, place your hand over the superficial ring (just above and medial to the pubic tubercle)

ASSESS THE SWELLING

Define its characteristics (see pages 26–28)	*?size* *?shape* *?fluctuant* *?transilluminable*

Press firmly over the
swelling/superficial ring

Ask patient to turn his/her
head away from you and cough

?expansile cough impulse

Ask patient to try to reduce the
hernia

He/she may request to lie down
to do this

While the hernia is still reduced,
place two fingers over the
deep ring (half-way between
pubic tubercle and ASIS)

Ask patient to cough
Watch

Release the pressure

*?hernia controlled by pressure
over deep ring* (indicates indirect
hernia)

Go to the other side of patient
Repeat the examination

COMPLETE THE EXAMINATION

Cover the patient up

Turn to the examiner

Ask to wash your hands

Present your findings

TYPICAL CASES

1. INGUINAL SWELLINGS AND HERNIAS

One way to remember the differential diagnosis of lumps in the groin is to think of the structures that normally lie in the region.

a. **Hernias**
- Inguinal (direct, indirect)
- Femoral

b. **Vascular structures**
- Saphena varix
- Femoral aneurysm

c. **Lymph nodes**
- Lymphadenopathy

d. **Muscle**
- Psoas abscess

e. **Hip joint**
- Psoas bursa

f. **Testis**
- Ectopic testis (in superficial inguinal pouch)
- Undescended testis (as it emerges from superficial ring)

g. **Spermatic cord**
- Lipoma of the cord
- Hydrocoele of the cord

Have a clear picture of the relation of these structures to the inguinal ligament:

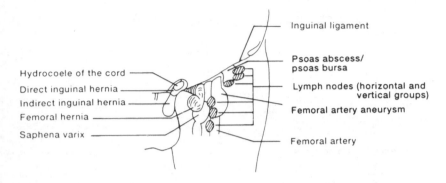

You may be asked what is meant by the term 'hernia'. The definition should roll off your tongue:

'The protrusion of the whole or part of a viscus, from its normal position, through an opening in the wall of its containing cavity.'

Another common question is: 'Why must a hernia be repaired?'

The answer is because of the potential complications of *obstruction* and *strangulation*. You should understand exactly what is meant by these two terms:

Obstruction: constriction at the neck of a hernial sac leads to obstruction of the loops of bowel within it.

Strangulation: constriction prevents venous return causing venous congestion, arterial occlusion and gangrene. This may lead to perforation causing peritonitis or a groin abscess.

Note that strangulation may occur without obstruction if only one wall of a viscus pouches into the sac ('Richter's hernia').

Case 1: Inguinal hernia

There is not much anatomy you need to know for finals.

However, a favourite question is to describe the anatomy of the inguinal canal: this is an intermuscular oblique passage 4 cm long. The following structures pass through it:

- Spermatic cord/round ligament
- Ilioinguinal nerve

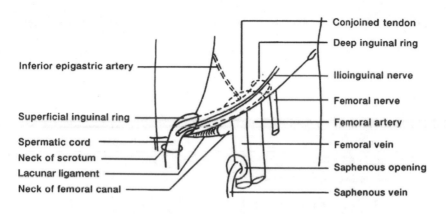

a. The walls

	ANTERIOR	POSTERIOR	FLOOR	ROOF
Medially	External oblique	Conjoined tendon	Inguinal ligament + Lacunar ligament	Conjoined tendon
Laterally	External + internal oblique	Fascia transversalis	Inguinal ligament	

b. The rings

(i) *External ring*
This is formed by the two crura of the external oblique aponeurosis (ie it is an opening in external oblique). It lies just above and medial to the pubic tubercle.

(ii) *Internal ring*
This is a U-shaped condensation of the fascia transversalis (ie it is an opening in the fascia transversalis).
It lies at the mid-point of the inguinal ligament. The inferior epigastric artery (branch of external iliac) runs *medially*.

Note the difference between the *mid-point of the inguinal ligament* (half-way between the ASIS and the pubic tubercle) and the *mid-inguinal point* (half-way between the ASIS and the pubic symphysis – landmark of the femoral pulse). The mid-point of the inguinal ligament lies 1–1.5 cm lateral to the mid-inguinal point.

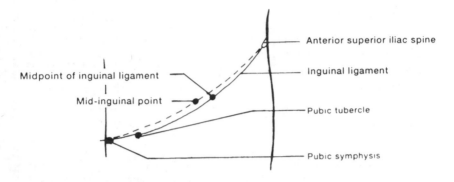

Understand the anatomy of direct and indirect hernias:

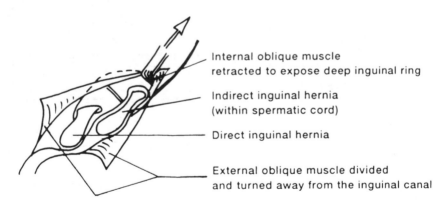

Some examiners are keen for you to be able to distinguish clinically between a direct and an indirect hernia:

	DIRECT	INDIRECT
Extends to scrotum?	No	Yes
Direction of reduction	Straight back	Up and lateral
Controlled by pressure over internal ring?	No	Yes
Direction of reappearance after reduction	Outwards to original position	Down and medial

Treatment: Surgical repair: herniotomy in the neonate and herniorrhaphy in children and adults. Initial attempts are made to reduce hernias that are not tender or accompanied by systemic problems, but obstruction and strangulation are treated as an emergency.

Case 2: Femoral hernia

You should know how to distinguish clinically a femoral from an inguinal hernia:

	INGUINAL HERNIA	FEMORAL HERNIA
Position relative to pubic tubercle	Superior and medial	Inferior and lateral*
Palpation	Soft	Firm: like bouncing a ball underwater
Percussion	May be resonant	Dull
Auscultation	Bowel sounds commonly heard	Bowel sounds rarely heard

*Note: Femoral hernias may bulge up into the groin crease (as shown on page 94).

Note the following additional points:

- In both men and women inguinal hernias are more common than femoral hernias. However, femoral hernias are more common in females than males.

- A femoral hernia is more likely to obstruct and strangulate than an inguinal hernia because of the narrow femoral ring. Furthermore, a femoral hernia is more likely than an inguinal hernia to strangulate without obstructing (Richter's hernia).

Revise the anatomy of the femoral canal:

Medially: lacunar ligament
Laterally: femoral vein
Supero-anteriorly: inguinal ligament
Inferoposterior: pectineal ligament of Astley Cooper over horizontal ramus of the pubis

Treatment: Femoral hernias have a narrow neck and are particularly prone to strangulation, possibly of the Richter variety. They therefore require early surgery and complications should be treated as an emergency. After inspecting the contents of the sac, ligating its neck and removing excess, repair is by suture of the inguinal ligament to the pectineal ligament whose fibres run along the superior ramus of the pubis. Two or three sutures are placed with a J shaped needle and ligated from medial to lateral to ensure that the femoral vein is neither damaged nor compressed.

The table below gives some of the clinical features of some other inguinal swellings.

	CONSIS-TENCY	COMPRESS-IBILITY?	COUGH IMPULSE?	OTHER FEATURES
Case 3: Saphena varix	Very soft	Yes	Yes	• Fluid thrill • Varicose veins
Case 4: Femoral aneurysm	Firm	No	No	• Expansile pulsation • Bruit
Case 5: Lymph node	Hard	No	No	• *Multiple* nodules • *Generalised* lymphadeno-pathy
Case 6: Psoas abscess	Soft	Yes	No	• Fluctuation between parts of abscess above and below inguinal ligament

Case 3 Treatment: A saphena varix is treated as part of varicose vein excision in symptomatic patients.

Case 4 Treatment: Femoral aneurysm is treated by surgical resection and replacement with a synthetic tube.

Case 5 Treatment: Lymph nodes may be part of a generalised infection. In localised infection the source must be identified and treated. Tuberculous nodes require treatment with a full course of antituberculous therapy. Primary and secondary malignant nodes require a tissue diagnosis. This is often possible through a fine needle aspiration, a full search being undertaken to identify a primary site, so that treatment of primary and secondaries can be planned.

Case 6 Treatment: Psoas abscesses are drained and appropriate antituberculous therapy initiated.

2. SCROTAL AND INGUINOSCROTAL SWELLINGS

It is unlikely you will be given a patient with a very tender swelling in an examination as this usually implies the following:

- Torsion of the testis: a surgical emergency
- Severe epididymo-orchitis: rare

A simplified diagnostic flowchart which excludes the latter two conditions is given below:

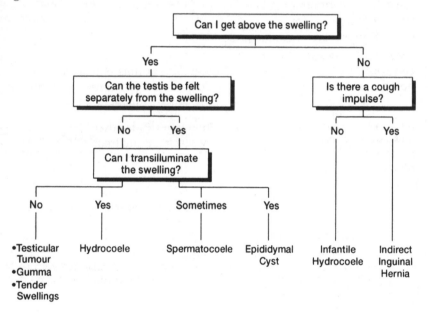

Case 7: Testicular tumour

This is an opaque mass, not felt discretely from the testis. It is usually painless but occasionally causes a dull ache. There is usually loss of sensation in the mass.

Remember that it may be associated with a secondary hydrocoele.

Note that lymphatic spread is along the site of its embryological origin, ie to para-aortic lymph nodes. It only spreads to inguinal nodes if the scrotum is invaded.

Investigation: The initial diagnosis is a clinical one. Tumour markers may be elevated – beta human chorionic gonadotropin (90% in teratoma, 25%

seminoma), alpha feto protein (50% in teratoma) plus alkaline phosphatase (50% in seminoma). CT is undertaken to identify para-aortic or mediastinal lymph nodes or secondaries in the liver or lungs.

Treatment: Orchidectomy via an inguinal approach. The testis is delivered through the incision in the external oblique and a vascular clamp applied to the spermatic cord, whilst a biopsy and frozen section are taken to confirm the diagnosis. A high ligation of the cord and orchidectomy is undertaken. Subsequent management depends on the stage and the pathology.

Stage 1: rising tumour markers post orchidectomy
Stage 2: abdominal nodes
Stage 3: supradiaphragmatic nodes
Stage 4: lung or liver metastases.

The subsequent treatment of testicular seminomas is radiotherapy for stages 1 and 2. Combination chemotherapy for stage 2 if nodes are greater than 5 cm and for cysts after radiotherapy, and for stages 3 and 4.

In teratoma, surgical resection of abdominal nodes is advocated as well as combination chemotherapy. Testicular lymphomas are treated by orchidectomy and chemotherapy.

Case 8: Varicocoele

This is a dilatation and elongation of the pampiniform plexus of veins, usually found on the left.

It feels like a 'bag of worms'.

It can only be felt with the patient standing.

Recent onset of a left-sided varicocele in an older man may be associated with a left renal cell carcinoma.

Treatment: In symptomatic enlargement of the pampiniform plexus and in the management of impotence, the plexus is excised preserving the testicular vein within the spermatic sheath, using an inguinal incision.

Case 9: Hydrocoele

This is a swelling that cannot be felt separately from the testis. It is fluctuant and transilluminable. It is due to excessive fluid collecting in the tunica vaginalis.

Understand the anatomy of the four types of hydrocoele. All of these come into your differential diagnosis of inguinal and inguino-scrotal lumps. A vaginal hydrocoele is by far the most common.

TYPE	AGE	COMMUNI-CATION WITH PERITONEAL CAVITY?	NOTE	DIAGRAM
a. Vaginal	All	No	May be *secondary* to underlying infection or a testicular tumour	
b. Congenital	child (aged < 3 yrs)	Yes	Main differential diagnosis is an indirect inguinal hernia: communicating orifice is too small for hernia to develop	
c. Infantile	All	No	Due to incomplete reabsorption of fluid from the tunica vaginalis after the processus vaginalis seals off	
d. Encysted hydrocoele of the cord	All	No	May occur anywhere along cord, causing a scrotal *or* inguinal lump	

Treatment: The hydrocoele may be secondary to trauma (haematocoele), infection or a tumour. Idiopathic hydrocoeles can be managed conservatively. Aspiration is possible although recurrence is usual. Definitive treatment is by surgical excision of the tunica vaginalis, or incision of the sac and radial plication sutures from within it to reduce its size.

Case 10: Epididymal cyst

Like a hydrocoele, this is brilliantly transilluminable. However, the testis can be felt separately.

Note that if it is filled with many sperm, it may be opaque. In this case, it is called a *spermatocoele*.

Treatment: Usually conservative but cysts may be excised if they are producing symptoms: care is taken not to damage surrounding structures as this may impair fertility.

Case 11: Absent testis in a child

Put your hand just lateral to the external ring and apply firm pressure downwards and medially. If you can 'milk' the testis down into the scrotum, the testis is *retractile*: descent is normal, but excessive cremasteric muscle activity in young children leads to the testis being drawn up.

Look carefully for other swellings in the area; there may be an *ectopic* testis. You may feel a lump in the following positions:

- Superficial inguinal pouch (superficial to external oblique and lateral to the pubic tubercle)
- Femoral canal (medial thigh)
- Perianally

Once you have *excluded* retractile and ectopic testes, you may diagnose an incompletely descended testis.

Remember to search for an inguinal hernia. This is present in 90% of cases of incompletely descended testes.

Treatment: Undescended testes usually descend into the scrotum by the age of two. Orchidopexy is undertaken after this age as (a) infertility is likely after puberty (b) the testes are more likely to undergo tortion and (c) the testes have a tenfold increased incidence of malignancy. The testes may lie in the inguinal canal or just above, (identification may be helped by CT). The spermatic vessels are preserved but other restricting tissues are excised to allow the testes to reach the scrotum. Ectopic testes are similarly mobilised and placed within the scrotum.

POPULAR VIVA QUESTIONS

1. Define 'hernia'.

2. Where might you find a hernia, other than the groin?

3. What anatomical factors can predispose to inguinal hernias?

4. What are the surface markings of the superficial inguinal ring/the deep inguinal ring?

5. Describe the anatomy of the inguinal canal.

6. Describe the anatomy of the femoral canal.

7. Why do we repair hernias?

8. What are the complications of hernias?

9. What is the difference between an indirect and a direct inguinal hernia?

10. Define the terms, 'herniotomy' and 'herniorrhaphy'.

11. What is the treatment of a strangulated inguinal hernia?

12. How would you manage a patient with a testicular tumour?

Answers on pages 182–185

11: Arterial insufficiency of the lower limb

THE HISTORY

'Arteriopath' patients are readily available for examinations because of their age and complications. They are usually given as long cases, as the histories tend to be extensive. In your 'history of presenting complaint', include not only the symptoms of peripheral vascular disease, but also all other symptoms, risk factors, past history and family history of cardiovascular and cerebrovascular and lower limb arterial disease.

Presenting symptoms

- Can you describe the pain in your legs? (Ask pain questions, see page 25)
- Does the pain come on when you walk/exercise?
- How far can you walk before you get the pain? (Claudication distance is best described in terms of a *known* distance, eg from the entrance of the hospital to the clinic)
- When you stop walking, how long does it take for the pain to go away?
- Can you walk *through* the pain?
- How long have you had the problem? Has it got any better or worse over this time?
- How does it affect your lifestyle?
- Have you any pain in your leg or foot at rest?
- What relieves your pain? (Rest pain may be relieved by walking about and hanging the leg over the side of the bed)

In a man, ask about erectile function (Leriche's syndrome).

Past surgical history

Ask about past operations and investigations for peripheral vascular disease. When you present your history, describe these events chronologically and as concisely as possible.

Past medical history

Ask about previous myocardial infarcts / strokes / transient ischaemic attacks.

Associated cardiovascular and cerebrovascular problems

Ask about chest pain / shortness of breath on exertion / palpitations / ankle swelling / loss of sensation or power of a limb / loss of vision / speech problems.

Risk factors

Ask about smoking / cholesterol levels / hypertension / diabetes.

Family history

Ask about a family history of cardiovascular / cerebrovascular / peripheral vascular disease.

Tailor the rest of your history towards the differential diagnosis. For example, it is important to ask about neurological symptoms, eg paraesthesia in the leg, as there may be a neurological cause of the pain.

THE EXAMINATION

The long case/OSLER

Pay particular attention to the following:

- Peripheral vascular system: look for ulcers on pressure areas and over the tips and between the toes. Record all pulses and bruits on a diagram (see page 108).
- Heart
- Fundoscopy
- Neurological examination of the lower limb: in a patient complaining of leg pain, you may be asked to explain how your examination findings point to a diagnosis of claudication/rest pain rather than nerve root pain.

The short case/OSCE

Listen carefully to or read the instruction: if your examiner asks you to examine the patient's lower limb, do not jump straight into the following scheme, but follow the systematic approach outlined on page 170. Similarly, if asked to examine an ulcer on a limb, proceed as for the examination of any ulcer (pages 29–30).

'Examine this patient's peripheral vascular system'

ACTION	NOTE	
Introduce yourself		
Ask permission to examine the patient		
Expose both legs completely		
LOOK		
Stand at the end of the bed and observe	Colour:	?white/blue/black
	Trophic changes:	?shiny skin ?hair loss ?loss of subcutaneous tissue ?ulcers
Look at pressure points: • lateral side of foot • head of 1st metatarsal • heel • malleoli	Ulcers: (pages 29–30)	?size ?shape/dimensions ?depth ?edge ?base
Observe: • tips of toes • between toes		

FEEL

Run the back of your hand
along both limbs
Compare both sides

?warm/cold
?point of temperature change

Press the tip of a nail for two
seconds
Count the number of seconds
for the nail to become pink again

?capillary refilling time

Feel pulses:

Compare right with left
In the long case/OSLER,
use a diagram to record pulses
and bruits:

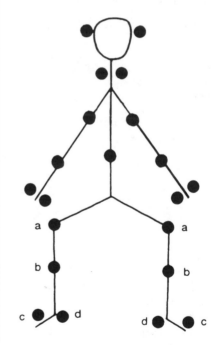

a. **Femoral pulse:** feel midway
   between symphysis pubis
   and ASIS (mid-inguinal
   point)

b. **Popliteal pulse:** ask the
   patient to bend his/her knee
   Put your thumbs on the
   tibial tuberosity and feel
   pulse with eight finger tips

c. **Dorsalis pedis:** feel along
   cleft between first two
   metatarsals
   Use three fingers

d. **Posterior tibial:** half-way
   along line between medial
   malleolus and the
   prominence of the heel

LISTEN

Listen for bruits at all sites,
ie along iliac, femoral and
popliteal arteries, and over the
adductor hiatus, on both sides

ASSESS FURTHER

Elevate leg about 15°
Look

?venous guttering

Elevate leg further

?angle at which leg becomes pale
(Buerger's angle)

Then ask patient to hang
leg over side of bed (Buerger's test)

?time of venous filling
?reactive hyperaemia on
dependency

SAY

'I would like to examine:
- the rest of the peripheral
  vascular system
- the heart
- the abdomen for an aortic
  aneurysm'

If asked to assess rest of
peripheral vascular system,

Feel:
- radial pulse
- carotid pulse

Listen for:
- carotid bruit
  (just behind angle
  of mandible)
- subclavian bruit
- radio-femoral delay

COMPLETE THE EXAMINATION

Make sure your patient is comfortable

Cover the legs

Turn to your examiner and present your findings

TYPICAL CASES

It is extremely unlikely that you will have a patient with an acutely ischaemic limb in the examination, as this is a surgical emergency. However, be aware of the causes of acute ischaemia and the symptoms and signs – remember the **6 P's:**

a. **P**ain
b. **P**araesthesia
c. **P**aralysis
d. **P**allor
e. **P**ulselessness
f. **P**erishingly cold

Case 1: Intermittent claudication

Don't worry if your history doesn't fit into any neat category: just report clearly and confidently on your findings. Ask yourself the following questions; this will help enormously in your presentation and discussion of the case with the examiners:

a. Is your patient's pain due to vascular disease?

It is quite possible that your patient has symptomless arterial disease with loss of pulses, but is suffering from a different cause of leg pain. Know the features of claudication pain:

- Cramp-like
- Felt in the muscle
- Comes on invariably and only with exercise
- Stops after about two minutes of rest

b. What is the differential diagnosis?

Think of the following:

(i) *Sciatica*
This is differentiated from claudication by the following features:

- History of disc lesion/back trouble
- Pain felt in back, down buttock and thigh
- No characteristic relationship to exercise
- Limited straight leg raising
- Neurological signs, eg wasting, loss of power, reflexes and sensation

(ii) *Osteoarthritis of the hip*
This can be difficult to distinguish as the pain is also worsened by exercise. The pain is felt in the hip joint but may be referred to the knee. It varies from day to day.

(iii) *Anterior tibial compartment syndrome* (rare in an examination)
This occurs in young people after unaccustomed exercise. The pain is felt in the anterior part of the lower leg.

(iv) *Cauda equina claudication*
This is the most difficult to distinguish. There are two pathologies. Both lead to sciatic-like pain and to limited straight leg raising after exercise.

- Disc pathology: partial compression of cauda equina by prolapsed disc
- Aorto-iliac disease: on exercise, a drop in pressure leads to ischaemia of cauda equina

c. What is the site of the main occlusion?

Try to relate your patient's symptoms (site of pain) and signs (absence of pulses, presence of bruits) to the anatomy. A mental picture of the angiogram helps:

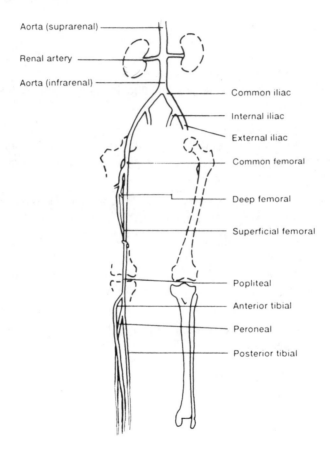

Aorta (suprarenal)

Renal artery

Aorta (infrarenal)

Common iliac

Internal iliac

External iliac

Common femoral

Deep femoral

Superficial femoral

Popliteal

Anterior tibial

Peroneal

Posterior tibial

Distinguish between femoro-distal disease and aorto-iliac disease:

	FEMORO-DISTAL DISEASE	AORTO-ILIAC DISEASE
Site of pain	● Calf	● Calf ● Thigh ● Buttock
Absent pulses	● Foot ● Popliteal	● Foot ● Popliteal ● Femoral

If aorto-iliac symptoms are unilateral, occlusion is probably of the common iliac artery. If symptoms are bilateral (rare), occlusion may be of the aorta. Think of the tetrad of Leriche's syndrome:

- Bilateral pain
- Impotence in male (no flow in internal iliac vessels)
- Bilateral absent femoral and distal pulses
- Aorto-iliac bruit

d. How severe is the claudication?

Your examiner will almost certainly ask how you would manage your patient. This is influenced by your assessment of the severity of your patient's claudication.

Use the following parameters:

- What is the claudication distance?
- Can your patient walk *through* the pain?
- How is it affecting your patient's lifestyle or work? (How far do they *need* to walk?)
- Has your patient tried conservative measures, eg stopping smoking, losing weight?
- How rapidly is the problem progressing?

Treatment: If patient can actively enjoy life, leave well alone; if not, consider arteriography and percutaneous dilatation.

∟ angioplasty
stenting

Case 2: Rest pain / critical ischaemia

The patient will usually be male, aged 60 +. A strong clue that he has rest pain is if his knee is bent or if his leg is hanging over the bed. Both these positions ease the pain.

The following features differentiate rest pain from claudication:

- The pain is distal, mainly in the toes and forefoot
- Skin pallor
- Trophic changes (page 107)
- Ischaemic ulceration at pressure points (page 37)
- Gangrene: usually dry and wrinkled
- Positive Buerger's test (page 109)

You may be asked why the pain particularly occurs at rest.

There are three reasons:

- Decreased arterial flow due to decreased assistance of gravity
- Physiological decreased cardiac output at rest
- Reactive dilatation of skin vessels to warmth (in bed)

Treatment: Pain needs to be managed. Arteriogram is used to assess whether it is possible to dilate arterial stenosis, whether surgical reconstruction is possible, and whether the patient is fit for surgery?

Case 3: Diabetic foot

As in the above case, your patient may have ulcers at pressure points and gangrenous toes. Remember that the pathology is multifactorial:

- Arterial occlusive disease
- Microscopic angiopathy
- Peripheral neuropathy (sensory, motor, autonomic)
- Infection

The following features distinguish the diabetic foot from the critically ischaemic foot:

- The patient is younger
- The foot is red and warm
- Gangrene is usually accompanied by infection: there may be deep collections of pus
- The pulses may be present

Treatment: Treat infection. May require conservative surgery to drain pus and remove dead tissue. May need more aggressive approach, as in Case 2.

Case 4: Aortic aneurysm

This is a common short and long case in surgical finals.

As always, look carefully. You may see a pulsating mass in the umbilical region.

An aortic aneurysm has an expansile pulsatility as opposed to a transmitted pulsatility. To distinguish between these, place the fingers of your two hands on either side of the mass and look to see if they are actually being pushed apart.

Measure the horizontal distance between your fingers: remember that, especially in thin females, the abdominal aorta is easily palpable.

Can your hand get above it? If so, it is infrarenal (most common).

Is the aneurysm tender? This suggests it may be about to rupture (a very unlikely examination situation!).

Auscultate over the swelling: a loud bruit (in the absence of a similar bruit in the heart) supports the diagnosis.

Check the femoral, popliteal and foot pulses. These are usually present, as patients presenting with aneurysms rarely have peripheral vascular disease. However, emboli from the aneurysm may cause distal occlusion. There may be an associated popliteal aneurysm.

Treatment: When the aneurysm is ≥ 6 cm across, the risk of rupture continues to rise; if the patient is otherwise fit, the aneurysm should be replaced with a synthetic tube, using percutaneous or surgical techniques.

Case 5: Amputation

Peripheral vascular disease is by far the commonest cause of amputation in the elderly. You may meet such a patient in the long case.

Take a detailed history of the immediate events leading up to the amputation but do not get bogged down in the probably lengthy history of previous operations such as bypasses and sympathectomies.

Your history should be geared largely towards the sociological implications of the amputation. Ask about mobility: can the patient climb stairs? Is he/she likely to be confined to a wheelchair existence? Assess the patient's ability to wash, dress and self care in other ways. Ask also about occupational therapy, home help, aids and appliances.

Determine whether the amputation is below knee/through knee/above knee and look carefully at the wound site. Is it infected? Are there contractures of the hip and knee joints?

Treatment: Vascular amputees need a wheelchair even where a prosthesis is proposed. Check whether their home needs adaptation: wheelchair accessibility is required for toilet and bathroom, reaching light switches, washing and cooking facilities, cupboards and getting onto their bed.

POPULAR VIVA QUESTIONS

1. Why does critical ischaemia lead to pain at rest?

2. What is the cause of a bruit?

3. What factors would influence your management of a patient with claudication?

4. What are the causes of diabetic foot disease?

5. What causes of intermittent claudication would you consider in a young patient?

6. What are the causes of an acutely ischaemic limb?

7. What are the symptoms and signs of an acutely ischaemic limb?

8. What is the ankle-brachial pressure index (ABPI)? Why measure it?

9. What anatomical features on the arteriogram determine the severity of ischaemia in an atherosclerotic limb?

10. What are the risk factors for peripheral vascular disease?

Answers on pages 185–186

12: Venous disorders of the lower limb

THE HISTORY

Include the following questions:

Presenting complaint

- What is your main problem? (The patient may be bothered by the appearance, aches and pains or something else.)
- Are you on your feet all day? Do your legs ache more towards the end of the day?
- How long have you had the problem? Have you seen anyone about it previously? Was it treated then?

Predisposing causes

- Does anyone else in your family have varicose veins?
- Have you ever been pregnant? Did you have any problems with your legs then? Did one leg swell up?
- Have you had any major injuries or operations? Did you have any problems with your legs then? Did one leg swell up?

In your systemic enquiry, ask about abdominal and gynaecological symptoms, particularly,

- Have your noticed any swelling of your abdomen?
- Have your clothes become tighter lately?

THE EXAMINATION

Venous insufficiency is a common short case. Practise the Tourniquet test. It may look easy on paper but the only way it doesn't end up an embarrassing fiasco in front of your examiners is for it to be a well-worn routine. Be absolutely clear about its significance. You may think you understand it but, with exam nerves, explaining it is another matter.

'Examine this patient's varicose veins'

ACTION	NOTE
Introduce yourself	
Ask permission to examine the patient	
Expose both legs with the patient standing up	
LOOK	
Compare shape of legs	*?beer-bottle leg*
Observe: • anteriorly • posteriorly	*?distribution of varicose veins*
Observe skin changes in 'gaiter area' (lower third of leg, especially above medial malleolus)	*?venous stars* → hair loss *?eczema* *?pigmentation* *?ulcers*
FEEL	
Run the back of your hand down both legs	*?warm over varicose veins*
Palpate along the medial side of the lower leg Ask if it is tender	*?tenderness* (occurs at sites of perforators)
Feel around the ankle	*?dermatoliposclerosis* *?pitting oedema*

Feel the saphenofemoral junction (4 cm below and lateral to pubic tubercle)	*?saphena varix*
Ask patient to cough	*?cough impulse* (indicates saphenofemoral incompetence)
Feel the saphenopopliteal junction (popliteal fossa)	
Ask patient to cough	*?cough impulse* (indicates saphenopopliteal incompetence)

(handwritten: thrill)

(handwritten: tapping test)

ASSESS FURTHER

a. Tap test
Place the fingers of one hand at the lower limit of a long varicose vein
Tap above with your other hand

?percussion impulse (indicates incompetence of *superficial* veins)

b. Tourniquet test
Ask patient to lie down flat

Elevate one leg until the superficial veins are emptied
Place a rubber tourniquet tightly around the upper thigh
(If patient is unable to hold up leg, ask the examiner to hold it up)

Ask patient to stand up
Watch *below* the tourniquet

?filling of superficial veins below tourniquet (indicates incompetent perforators *below* tourniquet)

Keep repeating the procedure, moving the tourniquet progressively down the leg

Position the tourniquet in between the sites of the perforator veins (see page 122)

Repeat until the veins *below* the tourniquet stay collapsed

Defines the segment of leg containing incompetent perforators

c. Trendelenburg test
Ask patient to lie flat
Elevate the leg until the superficial veins are emptied

Only perform this test if the tourniquet test is positive at upper third of thigh

Place two fingers at the saphenofemoral junction

Ask patient to stand up, keeping your fingers firmly in place
Watch leg

?no filling of superficial veins below fingers ?filling on release of finger pressure (indicates saphenofemoral incompetence)

d. Perthes' test
Place a tourniquet around the elevated leg so that the veins below tourniquet are empty

Ask patient to stand up and down on tip-toe ten times
Watch leg

?filling of superficial veins on exercise (indicates deep venous occlusion)

e. Listen
Auscultate over sites of marked venous clusters

?bruit (indicates AV malformation – rare)

SAY

'I would like to:
- examine the abdomen
- do a rectal examination
- do a pelvic examination (in females)
- examine the external genitalia (in males)'

?abdominal or pelvic mass (cause may be inferior vena caval obstruction)

**COMPLETE THE
EXAMINATION**

Lie the patient down

Cover the legs

Turn to your examiner and
present your findings

TYPICAL CASES

Although a patient with an acute deep vein thrombosis is unlikely to come
up in an examination, you should know about the presentation and differential diagnosis of this common emergency.

Be absolutely clear as to what is meant by the terms 'varicose veins' and
'venous insufficiency'. Your patient may have one or both of these conditions.

Case 1: Varicose veins

Your patient will usually have primary varicose veins, ie no known underlying cause. There may be a positive family history. However, always seek a
secondary cause (see history and examination above).

You may be asked to define varicose veins: these are 'dilated, tortuous,
thin walled, superficial veins'.

A knowledge of the anatomy will help in your description of the distribution of the varicosities. Note that the muscular wall usually prevents dilatation of the *main* leg veins: varicosities occur in the *tributaries*.

a. The long saphenous vein:

- Arises from the dorsal venous arch
- Runs anterior to the medial malleolus
- Runs behind the medial aspect of the knee
- Runs up the leg superficial to deep fascia
- Pierces cribriform fascia at the saphenous opening
- Empties into the femoral vein

b. The short saphenous vein:

- Arises from the dorsal venous arch
- Runs behind the lateral malleolus
- Runs up the midline of the calf superficial to deep fascia
- Pierces deep fascia over the popliteal fossa
- Empties into the popliteal vein

c. The perforator veins

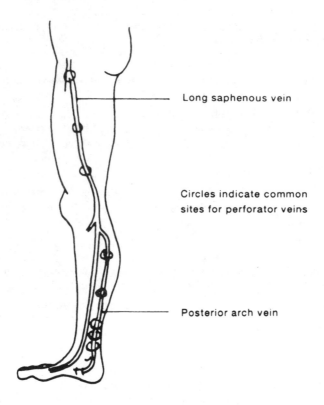

Long saphenous vein

Circles indicate common sites for perforator veins

Posterior arch vein

Treatment: Usually with the conservative measures of supportive hosiery and leg elevation. Uncontrolled symptoms: ligate saphenofemoral and other perforated sites, and inject or excise troublesome varicosities.

Case 2: Venous insufficiency

This describes the following dermatological course:

- Eczema (a low-grade cellulitis)
- Pigmentation (haemosiderin deposition) lipodermatosclerosis
- Venous ulcers (see page 36)

Your examiner will want to know if you have a clear understanding of the difference between *superficial* and *deep* venous insufficiency.

	SUPERFICIAL VENOUS INSUFFICIENCY	DEEP VENOUS INSUFFICIENCY
Aetiology	Primary varicose veins (unknown cause)	A late complication of deep vein thrombosis
Pathogenesis	Incompetent *perforator* veins: causes blood flow from *deep* to *superficial* system	Incompetent deep veins: leads to *raised pressure* in deep system. This causes blood flow from deep to *superficial* system (NB associated incompetent perforators may lead to *secondary* varicose veins)
Skin changes	Mild	Severe: 'beer-bottle leg' due to: • brawny oedema • dermatoliposclerosis (subcutaneous fat replaced by collagen)
Prognosis	Better response to surgery	Worse response to surgery

Treatment: Conservative measures, elevation of legs whenever convenient, supportive hosiery.

Case 3: AV malformations

Although AV malformations are rare, they are life-long problems often with good physical signs and they may therefore turn up as short cases.

Consider this diagnosis if you come across an easily compressible, superficial mass of vessels.

The malformation may be *congenital* or *acquired*. In a *congenital* AV malformation, your patient will tell you that the symptoms have been present from birth or childhood. There will often be gigantism of the affected limb. In *acquired* AV fistulae, there is a history of trauma. This may be surgically induced, as in the case of a fistula for haemodialysis.

Look for the following features:

- Signs of venous insufficiency
- Pulsatility
- Hum: always *listen* over large, unusually sited collections of varicosities

Treatment: Difficult as tend to recur: injection of sclerosant into centre of malformation, usually via an arterial catheter, however, if this is not possible, transcutaneously into (or smaller amounts around) the vessels. Surgical excision of localised malformation involving non-essential tissue, more aggressive management if the lesion is affecting vision or hearing, or if cosmetically unacceptable.

POPULAR VIVA QUESTIONS

1. Describe the aetiology of varicose veins.
2. What do you understand by the term venous insufficiency?
3. What are the indications for operating on a person with varicose veins?
4. How does an acute deep venous thrombosis present?
5. What are the causes of deep venous thrombosis?
6. What are the complications of a deep venous thrombosis?

Answers on pages 186–187

13: The hip

THE HISTORY

Pain

Ask the usual questions about pain (see page 25). Be clear as to where your patient's pain is felt *maximally* and where it *radiates*. Ask specifically if there is any knee pain.

When enquiring into exacerbating factors, ask about actions that load the joint, eg putting on socks, sitting in a low chair, rising from a sitting position and walking.

Stiffness

Ask if this is worse in the morning, on movement or after staying in one position.

Walking

- Ask how far the patient can walk.
- Has he/she noticed a limp or change in leg length?
- Ask in detail about aids and appliances: does the patient need a walking stick or a Zimmer frame?

In a long case, you must take a detailed social history. Find out how the problem affects the patient's life-style and whether it is deteriorating. Ask about the involvement of other joints: many patients with osteoarthritis or rheumatoid arthritis of the hip will have had other joint replacements.

THE EXAMINATION

The examination of the hip and knee is where most candidates let themselves down. You will probably not have had nearly as much practice as, say, examining an abdomen. Practise on each other: it is very easy for the examiner to see if you have done it before.

Most of the patients in short cases will have osteoarthritis and will be fairly fragile. If they are supine when you are introduced, it is probably simpler to start examining in this position. However, never forget to stand the patient up to perform the Trendelenburg test and to watch the gait.

In a long case, it is essential to examine the peripheral vascular system and to look for signs of infection in the leg. Both ischaemia and infection could potentially compromise a total hip replacement.

'Examine this patient's hip'

ACTION	NOTE
Introduce yourself	
Ask permission to examine the patient	
Expose both legs with the patient supine	
Check that the ASISs are at the same level	
LOOK	
Roll the patient to one side to observe the buttock and posterior thigh	skin: *?scars* *?sinuses*
	soft tissues: *?swelling* (the hip joint is deep and swelling is not usually seen)
	muscle: *?gluteal wasting*
Look at the ankles	bony alignment: *?obvious difference in leg length*
Look at the position of the patella and foot on each side	*?external rotation*
Look at the angle between the thigh and bed	*?fixed flexion deformity*

MEASURE

If there is a fixed deformity, place unaffected leg in the same position as the affected leg

Measure from the ASIS to the medial malleolus

?true leg lengths

Measure from the xiphisternum to the medial malleolus

?apparent leg lengths (see pages 134–135)

If there is any disparity in true leg length, ask the patient to bend the knees, keeping the ankles together

?shortening below knee (tibial shortening)

Compare the position of the two knees

?shortening above knee (femoral shortening)

If shortening is above the knee, put your thumbs on ASISs and feel down with your fingers until you reach the top of the greater trochanters

?Is there a difference in the distance between ASIS and greater trochanter (suggests shortening is in the hip joint itself)

FEEL

Ask if there is any tenderness

Palpate over greater trochanter

?tenderness

Palpate over anterior joint line (just lateral to femoral pulse)

Heat and swelling is only felt if patient is very thin

MOVE

a. **Thomas' test and flexion**
   Place your left hand in the hollow of the lumbar spine

see page 135

   Flex the hip and knee of the unaffected side until the lumbar spine straightens

?range of flexion of unaffected side (normally 130°)

Look to see if hip of the affected side lifts up from the bed

?*fixed flexion deformity of affected hip*

Flex the hip and knee of the affected side

?*range of flexion of affected hip*

b. **Abduction and adduction**
Rest your left forearm between the ASISs, keeping one hand on the pelvis

This stabilises the pelvis

Hold the ankle with the other hand

First abduct and then adduct leg until the pelvis starts to move

?*range of abduction* (normally 45°)
?*range of adduction* (normally 30°)

c. **Rotation**
Go to the end of the bed
Grasp the ankles and rotate each leg
internally and externally
Watch the patellae

Rotation may also be tested with the hip and knee flexed to 90°

?*range of internal and external rotation* (normally both 45°)

d. **Abnormal movement**
Alternately push and pull the leg along its long axis

?*telescoping* (a sign of marked instability)

STAND

Look again:

● anteriorly

?*rotational deformity*

● laterally

?*pelvic tilt*
?*increased lumbar lordosis*

● posteriorly

?*scoliosis*
?*gluteal wasting*

a. Trendelenburg test

Sit on a chair, facing the patient

Place one hand on each side of the patient's pelvis

The patient may rest his/her hands on your shoulders to maintain balance

Ask patient to stand on one leg

Feel if the hip on the *opposite* side rises or falls

?hip rises on opposite side (negative test – normal)

?hip falls on opposite side (positive test – abnormal: see page 133)

Repeat on the opposite side

b. Gait

Ask patient to walk away from you and then towards you Watch carefully

?Trendelenburg gait *?antalgic gait* *?supports, eg stick, frame*

COMPLETE THE EXAMINATION

Make sure patient is comfortable

Turn to the examiner

Present your findings

TYPICAL CASES

Case 1: Hip pain

If you meet a patient with a hip disorder in the long case/OSLER, he/she will almost certainly complain of pain.

You should know the characteristics of hip pain: this is usually felt maximally in the anterior groin. However, it is poorly defined and radiates variably to the following areas:

- Anterior thigh
- Lateral thigh

- Buttock
- Anterior knee
- Anterior lower leg

Remember that a patient with a primary hip disorder may present with isolated *knee* pain. This is because both the hip and knee contribute fibres to the obturator and femoral nerves.

Use the following table to differentiate hip pain from other local or distant causes:

	SITE OF MAXIMUM PAIN	RADIATION	EXACERBATING FACTORS
Hip pain	Anterior groin	Wide and variable (see above)	See history above
Trochanteric bursitis	Greater trochanter	Lateral thigh	Lying on affected side
Meralgia paraesthetica (entrapment of lateral cutaneous nerve of thigh)	Anterolateral thigh	None	• Pregnancy • Tight corsets • Jeans
Sacroiliac pain	Deep in buttock	Posterior thigh	Standing on one leg (affected side)
Nerve root pain due to prolapsed disc (Ll/L2)	• Groin • Back	None	Straining/ coughing
Ischaemic pain due to aorto-iliac disease (see page 113)	• Calf • Thigh • Buttock	None	Walking

Diagnosis: By clinical examination of the joints. Also assess for sensory and motor loss suggesting nerve damage. X-rays identify abnormalities of the

13: The hip

spine, pelvis and hip (important to compare the two sides), and are supplemented by images that identify soft tissue changes of the spine, pelvis and hip joint.

Treatment: This depends on identified cause of pain. Bursae can usually be treated conservatively until the inflammation subsides. Arthritic pain is managed by nonsteroidal anti-inflammatory drugs, although preferably not longterm. The lateral cutaneous nerve of the thigh should be released in meralgia paraesthetica. A protruded disc and peripheral vascular stenotic problems may require surgical management. Severe hip damage may require osteotomy, arthrodesis or prosthetic replacement. In all cases, consider physiotherapy, the use of a walking stick, and weight reduction.

Case 2: Abnormal gait

You may be asked to describe the gait of a patient with hip pathology.

The two main types are the **Antalgic** gait and the **Trendelenburg** gait (**waddling** gait if bilateral). You should know how they differ:

	ANTALGIC GAIT	TRENDELENBURG GAIT
Cause	Painful hip	Inefficient hip abduction
Weight-bearing/ stance phase	Shortened	Pelvis droops on opposite side
Direction to which body leans whilst weight-bearing	Towards affected side	Towards unaffected side

You may be asked to describe the mechanism of the Trendelenburg gait. This is probably best understood by considering the Trendelenburg test:

Normally, when standing on one leg, the abductors on the weight-bearing side contract so that the pelvis rises on the opposite side. A positive Trendelenburg test occurs when there is any inefficiency of hip abduction: the pelvis droops towards the unsupported side.

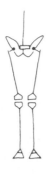
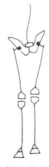
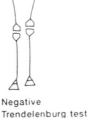
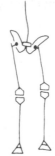

Negative
Trendelenburg test
(normal)

Positive
Trendelenburg test
(abnormal)

Inefficiency of hip abduction occurs as a result of the following:

a. Disturbance in the pivotal mechanism

(i) *dislocation* or *subluxation* of the hip
(ii) *shortening of the femoral neck*

b. Weakness of the hip abductors (gluteus medius and minimus)

(i) *myopathy* (usually bilateral)
(ii) *neuropathy* (L5 root lesion, usually unilateral)

Treatment: See Case 1.

Case 3: Arthritis of the hip

A patient with primary osteoarthritis of the hip is a very common short or long case. You could also be given a patient with rheumatoid arthritis and you should know how to distinguish the two conditions (see page 144). A patient with osteoarthritis will complain of hip pain (see Case 1). This will initially occur only after activity, but later be present at rest. Look carefully at the gait (see Case 2).

You may be asked the reasons why you measure apparent leg length and perform Thomas' test: arthritis may result in contractures which give rise to *deformities*. The most common are fixed *adduction* and *flexion deformities*. Both may be masked by compensatory movements.

The aim of measuring apparent leg length and performing Thomas' test is to unmask these contractures:

a. Apparent leg shortening

A fixed adduction deformity tends to cross the legs. Therefore, the pelvis compensates by tilting towards the affected side. This leads to apparent leg shortening.

(True shortening arises from loss of joint space.)

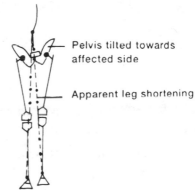

Pelvis tilted towards affected side

Apparent leg shortening

b. Thomas' test

A fixed flexion deformity can be completely masked by a lumbar lordosis. This is unmasked by performing Thomas' test.

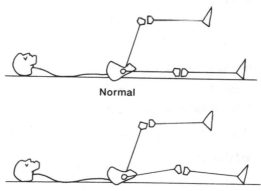

Normal

**Positive Thomas Test:
Flexion of normal hip reveals
fixed flexion of the other.**

Treatment: See Case 1.

POPULAR VIVA QUESTIONS

1. What are the risk factors for congenital dislocation of the hip?

2. How do we screen for congenital dislocation of the hip?

3. How would you manage a baby presenting with congenital dislocation of the hip?

4. What is a slipped upper femoral epiphysis?

5. What is Protrusio acetabuli?

6. What is Perthes' disease?

7. What is the difference between true and apparent leg shortening?

8. Describe the radiological appearances of osteoarthritis and rheumatoid arthritis.

9. How would you manage a patient with osteoarthritis of the hip?

10. What are the operations available for a patient with osteoarthritis of the hip?

11. What are the complications of a total hip replacement?

12. What are the contra-indications to a total hip replacement?

13. Describe Garden's classification of fractured neck of femur. What is its significance?

Answers on pages 187–189

14: The knee

THE HISTORY

If you have a patient with a knee complaint in the long case, bring out the following aspects in your presentation:

Pain

- Ask the usual questions about pain (see page 25).
- Be very clear as to whether the pain is generalised or localised.
- Tell the patient to point with one finger to where the pain is felt maximally.
- Ask if there is pain *above* the knee.
- Ask if it is exacerbated by walking or walking up and down stairs.

Stiffness

Ask if this is worse in the morning, on movement or after staying in one position.

Swelling

If preceded by an injury:
- Did the swelling occur straight away?
- Did the swelling occur after a few hours?

Episodes of locking or giving way

Explain to the patient exactly what you mean by these terms.
'Locking' is the sudden inability to extend the knee fully.
'Giving way' describes the feeling of apprehension on weight bearing.

THE EXAMINATION

As with the hip, examination of the knee will probably be relatively unfamiliar: practise on each other.

Don't worry too much about the 'additional assessment', eg the apprehension test and McMurray's test. Most of your examiners are not orthopaedic surgeons and just want to see that you have a basic routine of **LOOK, MEASURE, FEEL, MOVE.**

Never forget to ask to see the patient *walk* at the end of the examination. This will also give you the opportunity of looking at the popliteal fossa for posterior knee swellings.

'Examine this patient's knee'

ACTION	NOTE
Introduce yourself	
Ask permission to examine the patient	
Expose both legs with the patient lying down	
LOOK	
Compare the two sides	skin: ?erythema ?scars swelling: ?prepatellar ?infrapatellar
MEASURE	
Measure the circumference of each leg at a fixed point above the tibial tuberosity	Initial quadriceps wasting can be detected just medial to the upper part of the patella

FEEL

a. Temperature

Run the back of your hand
over both legs anteriorly and
down each side

?warm

b. Tests for effusion

(i) *Bulge test*

Positive with very *little* fluid
present

Empty the medial compartment
by massaging up the medial
side of the joint
Retain fluid in the suprapatellar
bursa with medial pressure from
one hand
Stroke down lateral side of the
joint with your other hand,
watching the medial side

*?appearance of ripple on
flattened medial surface*

(ii) *Patellar tap*

Positive with *large* effusion

Empty the suprapatellar bursa:
use your left hand to press
downwards and backwards
above the patella
Keep this hand in position
Push the patella sharply
back with your right hand

?feel/hear tap of patella on femur

c. Palpation of joint line

The joint line is lower than you
think

Bend the knee to about 50°
Palpate the *medial* joint line:
locate the tibial tuberosity and
move your finger medially and
proximally
Palpate firmly, anterior to
posterior
Ask if/when it hurts

tenderness: *?localised*
           ?generalised
synovium: *?thickened*
cartilage: *?swelling*

Palpate the *lateral* joint line
moving your finger laterally
and proximally from the tibial
tuberosity

Palpate the popliteal fossa   *?swelling*

MOVE

a. Flexion and extension
Ask patient to bend and then   range of active movement:
straighten his/her leg   *?limited flexion/extension*
Ask if/when it hurts

Place your hand over the
extended knee

Try to flex and extend the   range of passive movement:
knee joint yourself left hand   *?limited flexion/extension*
holding knee – and feeling for   *?crepitus*
crepitus – right holding lower leg

Try to hyperextend the   *?hyperextension*
leg by lifting the heel
upwards from the bed

b. Ligament stability
(i) *Medial collateral ligament*
Place one hand on the   *?excess movement*
lateral side of the *knee* and the
other on the *medial* side of
the ankle
Try to push the ankle laterally   *?pain*
while pushing the knee medially

(ii) *Lateral collateral ligament*
Place one hand on the *medial*   *?excess movement*
side of the *knee* and the other
on the *lateral* side of the *ankle*
Try to push the ankle medially   *?pain*
while pushing the knee laterally   *?gap sign* (opening up of lateral
                                      joint line)

(iii) *Anterior cruciate ligament*
Flex the knee to 90°
Steady foot by sitting close
(not on it)

Palpate the hamstrings to ensure
they are relaxed
Place thumbs of both your
hands on the tibial tuberosity
Grasp the lower leg and pull it
towards you

?tibia displaced anteriorly on femur
(positive anterior drawer sign)
There may be a false-positive
anterior drawer sign if the
posterior cruciate ligament is
ruptured

(iv) *Posterior cruciate ligament*
Repeat above test but push
the tibia *away* from you

*?tibia displaced posteriorly
on femur* (positive posterior
drawer sign)

ASSESS FURTHER

a. **The apprehension test**
Hold the patella laterally
with the knee extended
Bend the knee slowly

Only perform this test
if you suspect patellar instability

Watch patient's face

?resistance to further movement

b. **McMurray's test**
Flex the knee,
holding the joint steady

Only perform this test if
you suspect a torn meniscus

Use your other hand to slowly
extend the joint as you rotate
the foot first medially and
then laterally

?resistance to further movement
?pain
?click

STAND

Ask patient to stand up

Look from:
- in front
- the side
- the back

Ask patient to walk away from you and then towards you

COMPLETE THE EXAMINATION

Make sure patient is comfortable

Turn to the examiner

Present your findings

Genu valgum and varum are best seen in standing position

?genu valgum/varum
?genu recurvatum
?swelling in popliteal fossa

Gait: *?short-stepping*
?limp

TYPICAL CASES

As with the hip, pain is the most common presenting symptom. It may be associated with stiffness and mechanical problems.

1. KNEE PAIN

First ask yourself if the pain is due to knee pathology or if it is referred.

	KNEE PATHOLOGY	REFERRED PAIN
Localised?	Yes	No
Any pain above knee?	No	Yes
Exacerbated by walking?	Yes	No

Case 1: Anterior knee pain

Patellofemoral abnormalities cause anterior knee pain. This is characteristically exacerbated by:

- Going up and down stairs
- Sitting for a long time with the knee flexed

You may be asked the causes:

a. **Congenital** eg bipartite patella

b. **Injuries**

c. **Stress**
- Growth spurt (esp. adolescent females)
- Chondromalacia patellae (esp. adolescent males)
- Obesity
- Synovial shelf syndrome

d. **Bone osteochondritis**
- Osgood-Schlatter's/Sliding Larson's disease
- Osteochondritis dissecans

e. **Bursae and diverticulae**
- Bursitis
- Popliteal cyst/Baker's cysts

f. **Joint pathology**
- Rheumatoid arthritis
- Osteoarthritis
- Tuberculosis

Investigation: diagnosis can be made clinically but is confirmed radiologically, x-rays also demonstrate the extent of bone injury. MRI adds information on soft tissue disease, while arthroscopy allows both diagnosis and treatment of intra-articular problems.

Treatment: Fractures of the femoral and tibial condyles usually require internal fixation with aspiration of the joint and elevation, progressing to cast brace for early mobilisation. Traction may also be applied when osteoporosis is present. Undisplaced patellar fractures can be managed with a back-slab and mobilisation but displaced fractures may require wiring followed by a cast brace. Bursae and cysts: See Case 5; Popliteal aneurysms: See Case 6. Acute infection of the joint or adjacent osteomyelitis, are treated by urgent appropriate antibiotic therapy and may require aspiration of the joint or removal of bony sequestra. In tuberculous disease, a full drug course must be given. Subsequent management may include that of osteoarthritic changes. Osteoarthritis and rheumatoid arthritis are treated as summarised in Case 2.

Case 2: Arthritides

Compare and contrast the symptoms and signs of rheumatoid arthritis and osteoarthritis:

	OSTEOARTHRITIS	RHEUMATOID ARTHRITIS
Pain	+ +	+ +
Stiffness	+	+ +
Palpable synovium	–	+ +
Deformity	Genu varum	Genu valgum
Effusion	+	+ +
Limitation of movement	+ +	+ +
Crepitus	+ +	+ +
Joint instability	–	+

Ask specifically about the *pattern* of stiffness: this may tell you about the joint pathology:

	OSTEOARTHRITIS	RHEUMATOID ARTHRITIS
Morning stiffness	Sometimes	Very common
Time for morning stiffness to diminish	10 – 20 mins (approx)	30 mins – 1 hour (approx)
Stiffness after staying in one position	++	+

If you are asked to examine the knee in a short case, always glance at the hands. This will give you a clue if your patient has rheumatoid arthritis.

Remember: the knee may be the only joint involved in osteoarthritis whereas in rheumatoid arthritis, it is usually involved as part of a generalised syndrome.

Look carefully for scars of previous operations: your patient may have had a joint replacement. Look also at the thigh: note that, in all knee injuries there is rapid muscle wasting of the thigh muscles, particularly of the medial quadriceps.

Treatment: Osteoathritis of the knee is treated with analgesics and knee elastic support, progressing to depomedrone intra-articular injection and wash out of degenerative material. If symptoms progress, other measures may include patellectomy, tibial osteotomy, prosthetic joint replacement or arthrodesis. Treatment of rheumatoid arthritis involves treating the generalized disease and in the knee, arthroscopic synovectomy. When symptoms are not controlled by drugs supracondylar osteotomy is undertaken for marked valgus deformity and prosthetic joint replacement for extensive joint destruction. In both diseases, haemarthrosis and effusions are aspirated. Physiotherapy is an important aspect of rehabilitation.

Case 3: Mechanical problems

You would be extremely unlikely to have a patient with an acute injury in the examination. However, your patient could be a young man complaining of recurrent episodes of pain and locking following a meniscal tear.

Other causes of locking are plica syndrome (trapping of a synovial fold) and *loose bodies* (*'joint mice'*).

Know the causes of joint mice:

- Osteochondritis dissecans
- Synovial chondromalacia
- Osteochondral fracture
- Localised separation of articular cartilage

A knee 'gives way' in patellofemoral disease and when there is any weakness of the quadriceps, especially vastus medialis.

Treatment: When loose bodies or meniscal tears are present, arthroscopy allows diagnosis and treatment of the underlying problem, removing loose bodies and any damaged cartilage. If the anterior cruciate ligament requires replacement or repair for tears or knee instability, an above knee cast is required for six to eight weeks post-operatively.

Case 4: Knee deformities

You should know the causes of the two most common deformities, **genu valgum** and **genu varum**:

	GENU VARUM (BOW LEGS)	GENU VALGUM (KNOCK KNEES)
1. Physiological	Babies	Toddlers aged 3–4 (permissible to have 10 cm between ankles)
2. Arthritides	Osteoarthritis – cartilage loss in medial compartment	Rheumatoid arthritis
3. Metabolic	Vitamin C, D deficiency	Vitamin C, D deficiency
4. Growth disorders	• Paget's disease • Epiphyseal injury • Dysplasias, eg Blount's disease	• Epiphyseal injury • Dysplasias

Treatment: See Case 2.

2. KNEE SWELLINGS

Most lumps in and around the knee are due to bursitis or diverticulae. Know the differential diagnosis:

a. **Anterior** (rare)
- Pre-patellar bursa (Housemaid's knee)
- Infrapatellar bursa (Clergyman's knee)
- Osgood-Schlatter's disease

b. **Lateral/medial** (rare)
- Cyst of lateral meniscus
- Cyst of medial meniscus
- Exostosis

c. **Posterior**
- Semimembranous bursa
- Baker's cyst
- Popliteal aneurysm

You should be able to recognise a bursa by the following features:

- Not tender (unless infected)
- Smooth surface
- Fluctuant
- Transilluminable
- May be attached to skin
- Immobile

Case 5: Anterior knee swellings

a. **Pre-patellar bursitis: housemaid's knee**
Here the swelling is *over* the patella
Ask the patient his/her occupation: it is common in carpet layers, tilers and roofers, but not so common in housewives!

b. **Infrapatellar bursitis: clergyman's knee**
Here the swelling is distal to the patella

c. **Osgood-Schlatter's disease**
Suspect this condition in an adolescent who complains of pain after physical activity: look for a lump over the tibial tuberosity. On palpation, it is usually tender.

Treatment: Bursae and cysts are usually managed conservatively but may, if infected, need aspiration and appropriate antibiotics.

Case 6: Posterior knee swellings

a. Semimembranous bursitis

The swelling is behind the knee in the medial part of the popliteal fossa, above the joint line.

b. Baker's cyst/Popliteal cyst

This is a synovial diverticulum extending into the popliteal fossa through a deficit in the posterior capsule.
The swelling is behind the knee, below the joint line.

You may be asked to distinguish the terms 'popliteal cyst' and 'Baker's cyst':

Popliteal cyst:
- No underlying pathology
- Seen in young adults/children

Baker's cyst:
- Pathology of rest of knee, eg rheumatoid arthritis, osteoarthritis, gout, tuberculosis
- Often exacerbates pre-existing symptoms, eg further interference with knee flexion

c. Popliteal aneurysm

This is easily detected because of its expansile pulsation.
- Always palpate the other leg (it may be bilateral)
- Examine the peripheral pulses
- Palpate the abdomen for an associated aortic aneurysm

Treatment: Bursae and cysts (see Case 5). Popliteal aneurysms require surgical repair to prevent acute ischaemia from thrombosis or rupture.

POPULAR VIVA QUESTIONS

1. What is the normal angle of the femur on the tibia?

2. What are the causes of genu varum?

3. What are the causes of genu valgum?

4. What is the cause of Osgood-Schlatter's disease?

5. What is osteochondritis dissecans?

6. What are the causes of anterior knee pain?

7. What are the causes of 'a locked knee'?

8. What radiological features would you see in osteoarthritis?

9. What radiological features would you see in rheumatoid arthritis?

10. Where is the most common site for a meniscus to tear? How would such an injury present?

Answers on pages 189–190

15: The hand and foot

THE HISTORY

Hand and foot problems usually come up as short cases and OSCEs.
You may be told to ask the patient a few questions: first ask about the patient's main complaint. Then go through the usual questions about pain and swelling (page 25).

Ask specifically about loss of function:
* Can you hold a cup easily?
* Can you turn a doorknob?
* Do you have difficulty dressing yourself, eg doing up buttons?
* Do you have difficulty washing yourself?

THE EXAMINATION

The instruction will usually be to 'examine this person's hands'. Seek clues as to the underlying cause right from the beginning.

Look at the following:

* Elbows: ?*rheumatoid nodules*   — psoriasis
* Nails and skin: ?*nail pitting* ?*psoriasis*
* Ears: ?*gouty tophi*

'Examine this patient's hand(s)'

ACTION	NOTE
Introduce yourself	
Ask permission to examine the patient	
Place a pillow on the patient's lap and tell the patient to rest *both* hands on it	

LOOK

Observe:
dorsal surface

long term damad *JIR*

* *loss of alignment*
* *scar*
* *symmetrical or asy*

skin: ?thin/bruised *praximin*
nails: ?clubbing/pitting
muscle: ?wasting of dorsal interossei
joints: ?swelling
(Heberden's or Bouchard's nodes)
bony deformities:
?rheumatoid arthritis
(page 159)

palmar surface

scar from carpal tunnel release

skin: ?erythema
?Dupuytren's contracture

muscles: ?wasting of thenar/hypothenar eminence and ventral interossei

from the side
(patient's hands outstretched)

?finger drop

knuckles (patient's fists clenched)

a Garrod's pad
?swelling of MCP joints

hands in praying position
and back to back

Examine bulk of thenar and hypothenar eminences:
?same on both sides

FEEL — *for peripheral pulses, muscle bulk, palmar tender thickening*

Ask if hands are painful

Run the back of your hand
over patient's forearm and fingers
Compare the temperature of
both sides

?warm/warmer

Squeeze gently and palpate over:
- MCP joints 2–5
- IP joints 2–5

watch patient face

?areas of maximum tenderness
?soft tissue swelling
?bony swelling

Bimanual examination — mcp
— BIJ
— PIJ
— wrist.

Squeeze gently and palpate over:
- thumb joints
- radiocarpal joint
- inferior radioulnar joint

?areas of maximum tenderness
?soft tissue swelling
?bony swelling

MOVE

Place your thumb on patient's palm and move each MCP and IP joint in turn

?limited range of movement
?crepitus from flexor tendon

TEST POWER

Ask patient to grip two of your fingers as hard as possible

?strength of power grip

Ask patient to oppose thumb to index finger as hard as possible
Hook your index finger under point of contact
Try to pull it through

?strength of precision grip

Test thumb abduction:
'Point your thumb up towards your nose. Now keep it there and don't let me push it downwards'

?strength of abductor pollicis longus (median nerve)

Test finger abduction:
'Spread your fingers wide apart. Don't let me push them together'

?strength of interossei (ulnar nerve)

Test finger adduction:
'Grip this sheet of paper between two fingers at a time'

?strength of interossei (ulnar nerve)

TEST SENSATION

Compare sensation on each side with a pinprick over:
- index finger
- little finger
- lateral aspect of thumb base

median nerve
ulnar nerve
radial nerve

ASSESS FUNCTION

Ask patient to undo a button

Ask patient to write his/her name

ASSESS FURTHER	Only perform the following tests if appropriate

If you suspect ulnar nerve lesion:

Froment's sign	
Ask patient to grasp a piece of paper between the thumb and index finger (using both hands) Try to pull paper away	*?flexing of terminal phalanx as you pull away* (flexor pollicis brevis compensating for weak adductor pollicisbrevis-ulnar nerve)

If you suspect carpal tunnel syndrome:

a. **Tinel's sign** Percuss over the distal skin crease of wrist	*?pain/tingling felt over lateral palm*
b. **Phalen's test** – 60 second. Hold the patient's wrist maximally flexed for one minute	*?pain/tingling felt over lateral palm*

If patient cannot flex an IP joint:

Hold middle phalanx still Flex distal phalanx Hold all fingers down except the one to be tested Tell patient to flex that finger	*?flexion present* (indicates flexor digitorum superficialis intact)

If you suspect de Quervain's tenosynovitis:

Finkelstein's test Tell patient to grasp his/her thumb in the adjacent palm Now deviate the fist towards the ulnar side	*?pain* (indicates de Quervain's tenosynovitis)

If you are asked to examine a patient's foot, follow the usual routine of 'LOOK, FEEL, MOVE', examining each joint in turn as outlined on page 171. There will usually be an obvious abnormality which you should describe systematically before giving your diagnosis.

TYPICAL CASES

1. THE HAND

Case 1: Contracted hand

You may be shown a contracted hand. Your differential diagnosis will include an ulnar nerve palsy (page 157) and Klumpke's palsy (page 157) which both result in a clawed hand. A contracted hand may result from the following conditions:

	CAUSE	JOINTS AFFECTED
Dupuytren's contracture	● Autosomal dominant inheritance ● Alcohol/cirrhosis ● Phenytoin ● Diabetes mellitus ● AIDS, tuberculosis	*Flexion* of MCP and PIP joints (affects ring and little fingers)
Volkmann's contracture	Trauma at/below elbow leads to ischaemia of forearm muscles	*Flexion* of MCP and IP joints. Can be straightened only when wrist is flexed
Shortening of intrinsic hand muscles	● Spasticity ● Scarring due to trauma/infection	*Flexion* of MCP joints *Extension* of IP joints *Adduction* of thumb

The most common cause of a contracted hand is **Dupuytren's contracture**:

- Feel for the hard, subcutaneous nodules on the palmer surface
- Look at the knuckles which may also be thickened (Garrod's pads)
- Look at the other hand
- Ask to examine the soles of the feet: similar nodules may be felt

If permitted, ask the following questions to determine the cause:

- Do you drink alcohol? How much per day?
- Do you have diabetes?
- Do you suffer from epilepsy? Are you on phenytoin?

Treatment: Dupuytren's contracture is usually managed conservatively but where there is progressive flexion of ring and middle fingers, the thickened fascia may be excised with splintage for six weeks post-operatively. In severe, persisting, disabling deformity, the little finger may be amputated.

Volkmann's contracture and shortening of the intrinsic hand muscles are usually managed conservatively although muscle release procedures and tendon transfers may be possible.

Case 2: Median nerve lesion

This is usually carpal tunnel syndrome.

You may be asked the associations. Classify your answer:

- Endocrine causes (acromegaly, myxoedema)
- Connective tissue diseases (rheumatoid arthritis)
- Fluid retention (congestive cardiac failure, pregnancy)
- Trauma

Remember the signs:
a. Sensory loss: over lateral three and a half digits:
    Note that the palm may be spared as the palmar branch of median nerve passes superficial to the flexor retinaculum.

b. Motor loss and wasting: affects **LOAF**:
    Lumbricals (lateral two)
    Opponens pollicis
    Abductor pollicis brevis (easiest to detect)
    Flexor pollicis brevis

c. *Positive Tinel's sign and Phalen's Test* (see examination scheme, page 154)

Treatment: See Case 6.

Case 3: Ulnar nerve palsy

This is usually due to trauma at the elbow: *look* for scars here.

It may occasionally arise from repeated trauma to the heel of the hand, in which case there is no sensory loss.

Revise the signs:
a. **Position:** claw hand
b. **Sensory loss:** over little and ring fingers
c. **Motor loss and wasting:** affects the interossei; most noticeable dorsally. There is weakened finger abduction and adduction
d. **Positive Froment's sign** (see page 154)

Treatment: See Case 6.

Case 4: Radial nerve palsy

The commonest cause is when the patient falls asleep with his/her arm hanging over the edge of the chair ('Saturday Night Palsy'). Remember that the radial nerve lies in the spiral groove and can therefore also be damaged by fractures of the shaft of the humerus.

The main signs are wrist drop and wasting of the posterior forearm muscles. There is very little sensory loss: only over the anatomical snuffbox.

Treatment: See Case 6.

Case 5: Erb's palsy (C5 C6 roots)

The most common causes are birth trauma and injury. The signs are as follows:
a. **Position:** arm internally rotated with the forearm pronated and the palm facing backwards (the waiter's tip sign)

b. **Sensory loss:** over deltoid

c. **Muscle weakness and wasting:** affects deltoid, most of shoulder rotator muscles, biceps and brachioradialis

d. **Reflexes:** absent biceps and supinator reflexes

Treatment: See Case 6.

Case 6: Klumpke's palsy (T1 root)

This may be caused by a cervical rib or apical lung tumour (Pancoast's tumour): remember to check for an associated Horner's syndrome – meiosis, ptosis, enophthalmos and anhidrosis.

The hand is clawed and wasted. There is sensory loss over the inner aspect of the arm and forearm.

Treatment: Where the nerve injury is neuropraxia, there may be some spontaneous recovery. For more severe injuries, the site of damage must be identified and immediate repair may be possible. Recovery is more likely in children and in pure motor or sensory nerves. Brachial plexus injuries involving avulsion of the nerve roots are not amenable to surgery and a useless, flail upper limb is an occasional indication for amputation. Progress of healing can be followed by a positive Tinel's sign.

Case 7: Dropped finger

● Usually affects little and ring fingers Finger can be passively extended but drops down upon release

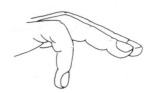

Cause: Extensor tendon rupture (close to ulnar styloid)

Treatment: Tendon repair

Case 8: Mallet finger

● Terminal IP joint cannot be extended

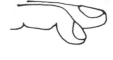

Cause: Division/avulsion of extensor digitorum longus (at base of distal phalanx)

Treatment: A splint in the acute phase, retaining hyperextension of the distal interphalangeal joint. Old injuries with marked deformity may require tendon reconstruction

Case 9: Boutonnière's deformity

● Flexion of PIP joint
● Hyperextension of DIP joint

Cause: Rupture of central slip of extensor expansion. Associated with rheumatoid arthritis

Treatment: Surgical correction by transferring the lateral slip of the tendon to the middle phalanx

Case 10: Swan neck deformity
(opposite of Boutonnière's deformity)

- Hyperextension of PIP joint
- Flexion of DIP joint

Cause: Associated with rheumatoid arthritis

Treatment: Painful deformed and defective hands may be improved by synovectomy with or without prosthetic replacement of the metacarpophalangeal and interphalangeal joints

Case 11: Trigger finger/ Stenosing tenosynovitis

- Patient's finger clicks when it is bent
- When patient straightens out hand, affected finger remains bent and then straightens with a click
- Feel for a tender nodule over the tendon sheath

Cause: Inflammatory thickening of the tendon or its sheath

Treatment: The stenotic area of the tendon sheath is incised to release and allow free movement of the tendon.

Case 12: Rheumatoid arthritis

This is a very common short case. You should be able to describe the characteristic deformities:

- Ulnar deviation of the fingers
- Boutonniere's deformity
- Swan neck deformity
- Z-deformity of the thumb
- Subluxation of the MCP joints
- Dorsal subluxation of the ulna at the carpal joint

Also look for the following additional features:

- Swelling of the PIP joints
- Wasting of the small hand muscles
- Atrophic skin and purpura (secondary to steroid therapy)

Palpate the elbows for rheumatoid nodules.

Treatment: Painful deformed and defective hands may be improved by synovectomy with or without prosthetic replacement of the metacarpophalangeal and interphalangeal joints.

Case 13: Osteoarthritis

Note especially:

- Heberden's nodes: bony thickening of DIP joints
- Bouchard's nodes: bony thickening of the PIP joints
- Squaring of thumb: involvement of carpometacarpal joint of thumb

Treatment: conservative management.

Case 14: The wasted hand

This is a common short case.

The two most common causes of generalised hand wasting are old age and rheumatoid arthritis.

However, remember neurological causes:

- Palpate for a cervical rib
- Look for scars around the elbow (ulnar nerve palsy)
- Test abductor pollicis brevis and the interossei for median and ulnar nerve palsies respectively

Treatment: If a T1 nerve injury is identified, the offending cervical rib or compressing band must be removed or released surgically as soon as possible.

2. DISORDERS OF THE FOOT

The three common foot problems you will see in an examination are hallux valgus, hammer toe and claw toes.

Case 15: Hallux valgus 'bunions'

This condition is usually bilateral: always look at the other foot. Examine for the following features:

- Inflammation: heat and redness over the bunion
- Associated hammer toe
- Corns and callosities over and under the metatarsal heads
- Secondary osteoarthritis of the metatarsophalangeal joint

Treatment: Excision of the prominent head of the metatarsal with or without corrective osteotomy, and reconstruction of the joint. Alternatively the joint may be excised or arthrodesed.

Case 16: Hammer toe

This usually affects the second toe. It may be bilateral. There is a fixed flexion deformity of the PIP joint.

Treatment: See Case 17.

Case 17: Claw toes

Claw toes are usually idiopathic. However, you should know the secondary causes:

- Rheumatoid arthritis
- Neurological problems, eg polio, Charcot-Marie-Tooth disease, diabetes

Look for an associated pes cavus (high foot arch).

Treatment: These deformities are usually managed conservatively with appropriate footwear but the affected joints may be arthrodesed.

POPULAR VIVA QUESTIONS

1. THE HAND

1. What muscles do the median, ulnar and radial nerves supply in the hand?
2. What are the signs of median, ulnar and radial nerve palsies?
3. What are the causes of median, ulnar and radial nerve palsies?
4. In what position would you fix the hand after injury to avoid stiffness?
5. What is de Quervain's tenosynovitis?
6. What is a trigger finger?
7. What associations of Dupuytren's contracture do you know?

2. THE FOOT

1. Describe the deformity of club foot.
2. Are there any indications for treating flat feet?
3   What is hallux valgus? How would you manage it?
4. What is the difference between hallux valgus and hallux rigidus?
5. What are the causes of pes cavus and claw toes?

Answers on pages 190–192

16: The post-operative patient

Surgical wards have a high proportion of post-operative patients who are readily available for examinations. Patients who have recently undergone vascular, gastro-intestinal or transplant surgery may come up as long cases.

In any part of the clinical examination, expect questions on post-operative complications (eg pain, respiratory problems, wounds) and fluid balance. Familiarise yourself with bedside charts which may be used as a basis for discussion and OSCEs.

THE HISTORY

Take a history of both the presenting complaint (ie circumstances that led up to this admission) and post-operative events. Screen for common post-operative complications by asking the following questions:

Pain

- Are you in any pain? (Ask specifically about leg pain, chest pain and increasing wound pain)

Respiratory symptoms

- Since the operation, have you:
  - been short of breath? ~ SOB
  - had a cough?
  - coughed up blood?

Gastrointestinal symptoms

- Have you passed a motion or flatus since the operation?
- Have you noticed any swelling of your abdomen?
- How is your appetite?

- Are you able to eat normally?
- Do you have any nausea or vomiting?

Urinary symptoms

- Did you have a catheter?
- Have you passed urine since the operation?
- Have you had any difficulty passing urine?
- Is there any pain when you pass urine?

Ask also about drugs, including analgesics, antibiotics and heparin prophylaxis.

Take a detailed social history: does the patient live alone? Who will look after him/her after leaving hospital? On which floor does the patient live: are there many stairs to climb/do the lifts work?

THE EXAMINATION

When you examine a post-operative patient, first take a note of the tubes and measuring devices around the bed. Then go on to examine the patient. Finally, never omit to look at observation, fluid and drug charts which will probably be available.

Follow the scheme below:

'Examine this post-operative patient'

ACTION	NOTE
LOOK AROUND THE BED	
• Drips	*?number*
	?sites
	?fluid type
	?rate of delivery
• Lines	*?central venous line*
	?arterial line

- Drains

  ?number
  ?site
  bag contents: ?*amount*
  ?*colour*
  ?*blood*

  seal: ?*sealed unit*
  ?*underwater seal*

- Nasogastric tube

  bag contents: ?*amount*
  ?*colour*

- Urinary catheter

  ?*open bag*
  ?*wash-out attachment*
  ?*volume of urine*
  ?*blood in urine*

EXAMINE PATIENT

a. Preliminary assessment
Form a general impression
of the patient

?*ill*
?*in pain*
?*evidence of recent weight loss*
?*hydration status*

Check the mental state

?*orientated in time/place/person*

Look at the hands

?*pale skin creases*
(clinically anaemic)
?*muscle wasting*
?*loss of skin turgidity back of hand*
(dehydration)

Take the pulse

Take the blood pressure

Look at the eyes

?*sunken* (dehydration)

Look at the conjunctivae

?*pale* (clinically anaemic)

Look at the sclerae

?*jaundice*

Pinch skin on abdomen

?*lack of skin turgor* (dehydration)

feve

b. Examine the chest
   (refer also to medical text)

signs of: ?*infection* → *pain*
            ?*atelectasis* *SOB*
            ?*fluid overload*
            ?*dehydration*

c. Examine the abdomen
   (pages 72–75)

Ileus may lead to absent
bowel sounds after abdominal
or retroperitoneal surgery

d. Examine the wound

?*site*
?*type*
?*stitches/clips*
?*apposition of edges*
?*redness*
?*swelling*
?*bruising*
?*discharge*

e. Examine the legs

?*swelling*
?*tenderness over calf*

f. Examine the pressure areas:
   ● sacrum
   ● heels
   ● elbows

?*bedsores*

LOOK AT THE CHARTS

temperature chart

?*pyrexia*

nursing observations

?*pulse*
?*blood pressure*
?*respiratory rate*

fluid balance

?*input = output*

drug chart

?*type of analgesia*
?*drugs for medical problems*

COMPLETE THE EXAMINATION

Make sure your patient is comfortable

Turn to the examiner and present your findings

POPULAR VIVA QUESTIONS

2.5-3L   70mmol   60mmol

1. What is the normal daily requirement of water, sodium and potassium?

2. How would you determine the amount of fluid to prescribe in the first 24 hours after a laparotomy?

3. How would you assess dehydration/overhydration?

4. What is the difference between a crystalloid and a colloid?

5. What are the complications of blood transfusion?

6. Define oliguria.

7. How would you manage a patient with oliguria for more than 24 hours post-operatively?

8. How would you manage a patient with an increased pulse rate and drop in blood pressure post-operatively?

9. Tell me about prophylaxis against deep vein thrombosis.

10. What are the possible causes of a pyrexia between two and ten days post surgery?

11. What are some of the alternatives for pain relief post surgery?

12. What are some of the predisposing factors for wound infection?

13. What are the respiratory complications after major surgery?

14. How would you manage a patient with (a) insulin-dependent and (b) non-insulin-dependent diabetes pre-, peri-, and post-operatively?

Answers on pages 192–195

17: General approaches

Most of this book is devoted to specific systems or parts of the body. This chapter gives examination schemes which are applicable to more than one system.

Included are approaches to 'a *limb*' and '*a joint*'.

A LIMB

You may be told to examine a limb, with no clues from the examiner as to which system is abnormal. Always approach the problem by looking systematically and remarking on any abnormalities you see. Then go on to examine the appropriate systems.

The scheme on the following page gives one approach to examining a leg.

'Examine this patient's leg'

ACTION	NOTE
LOOK	skin: ?*varicose veins/signs of venous insufficiency* (121–124) *Trophic changes/ ischaemic ulceration/ gangrene* (107)
	soft tissues: ?*swelling of knee* (146–148) ?*quadriceps wasting* (138) ?*gluteal wasting* (128)
	bony alignment: ?*genu varum/ valgum* (146) ?*disparity in leg length* (134)

FEEL

Feel pulses

Check for lymphadenopathy

MOVE

Check active and passive movement of each joint

Feel for crepitus

NEUROLOGICAL ASSESSMENT

Test response to light touch (using cotton wool)

Test response to a pin-prick

A JOINT

The most common orthopaedic long and short cases are hips and knees. However, do not panic if you are given a shoulder, an elbow, an ankle or a back to examine. Follow the same routine for all joints:

'Examine this patient's joint'

ACTION	NOTE
LOOK	skin: *?erythema* *?scars* *?sinuses*
	soft tissue: *?swelling*
	muscle: *?wasting*
	bony alignment: *?deformity*
FEEL	
Ask if there is any tenderness	
Run the back of your hand over joint	temperature: *?warm*
Feel any swelling	swelling: *?fluid* *?soft tissue* *?bony*
Feel over the joint line	*?tenderness*
MOVE	
Ask patient to move the joint in each direction in turn	*?range of active movement*
Move joint in all directions, feeling for crepitus	*?range of passive movement* *?crepitus*

Viva answers

CHAPTER 6: PAIN, SWELLING AND ULCERS

1. See examination section pages 26–30.

2. A boil is an abscess in a superficial hair follicle. In a carbuncle, the infection has extended into the subcutaneous tissue and it may be a collection of subcutaneous abscesses with or without external tracts.

3. A hypertrophic scar resolves within six months. Keloids extend into the surrounding tissues and recur after surgery. One or more steroid injections may help. Keloids are more common in Afro-Caribbean people.

4. Itching, colour change, increase in size, ulceration, bleeding, halo of pigmentation, satellite nodules, enlarged local lymph nodes and distant spread.

5. Basal cell carcinoma has a smooth rounded pink pearly edge; squamous cell carcinoma has an irregular raised everted red-brown edge.

6. Age, sunlight, ionising radiation and chemicals, such as soot, dyes and tar.

CHAPTER 7: NECK SWELLING AND THYROID LUMPS

1. (a) Infection: from the skin of the head and neck, the tonsils, adenoids and throat, and other sites in the ear and nose, paranasal air sinuses, pharynx and larynx. (b) Part of generalised lymphadenopathy: acute (e.g. infectious mononucleosis, cytomegalovirus) or chronic (e.g. TB, brucellosis, secondary syphilis, HIV). (c) Malignancy: primary (e.g. lymphoma, Hodgkin's and leukaemias) or secondary (e.g. metastases from carcinoma of the head and neck, breast, chest and abdomen). (d) Amyloid and sarcoid infiltration.

2. The anterior triangle lies anterior to the sternomastoid muscle below the mandible. The triangles from each side meet in the midline. Lymph nodes and abscesses such as tuberculous. Salivary glands (submandibular and parotid), carotid body tumours, carotid aneurysms, branchial cysts and tumours of the sternomastoid.

Midline swellings may appear in either anterior triangle, including thyroid swellings, thryoglossal cysts, sublingual dermoid cyst, plunging ranula, pharyngeal pouch, subhyoid bursa, and in carcinomas of the larynx, trachea and oesophagus.

3. Physiological enlargement at puberty and pregnancy; simple and multiple colloid that may be associated with goitrogens; dyshormogenesis; iodine deficiency; autoimmune thyroid disease (Hashimoto's thyroiditis and Grave's disease); other thyroid disease (DeQuervain's and Riedel's); tumours: benign and malignant (primary or secondary); tuberculosis; sarcoidosis.

4. **Hyperthyroidism**: Grave's disease (autoimmune; younger patients with diffusely enlarged goitre and bruit), multinodular goitre (in older patients), toxic adenoma and excessive thyroxin replacement. Rare causes: metastatic thyroid carcinoma, TSH secreting pituitary tumour, chorionocarcinoma, hydatidiform mole and neonatal thyrotoxicosis. **Hypothyroidism**: primary myxodema (autoimmune; older patients with no goitre), Hashimoto's thyroiditis, over-zealous treatment with drugs, surgery or radioiodine. Neonatal cases: agenesis or maternal antithyroid agents.

5. Failure of medical treatment; retro-sternal extension and tracheal compression; symptoms of multinodular enlargement. Note that surgical treatment is safest in the midtrimester of pregnancy.

6. Continuation of long term carbimozole or other antithyroid agents; additional propranolol in severe cases and uncontrolled cardiovascular symptoms; Lugol's iodine two weeks preoperatively.

7. Immediate complications: acute tracheal obstruction from haematoma, thyroid crisis, recurrent laryngeal nerve damage. Longer-term complications: hypocalcaemia from parathyroid excision, long-term hypothyroidism and recurrent hyperthyroidism.

8. Papillary and follicular carcinoma, medullary carcinoma (associated with multiple endocrine neoplasia IIa and IIb), anaplastic carcinoma and aggressive neoplasm (of middle age and elderly patients), and malignant lymphomas (associated with longstanding Hashimoto's thyroiditis).

9. Submandibular: in the floor of the mouth on the submandibular papilla situated on each side of the frenulum of the tongue. Parotid: opposite the crown of the second upper molar tooth

10. Stenosis in the duct due to chronic infection and oral disease around the papilla. They usually occur in the submandibular gland leading to pain and distention on eating; very rarely in the parotid gland.

11. Pleomorphic adedoma. Small nonprogressive tumours: observation. Others: superficial parotidectomy or excision with a surrounding cuff of normal tissue. The more extensive excision requires particular care of the facial nerve. Occasionally radiotherapy is required for recurrent problems.

12. Benign: smooth, lobulated painless, may be bilateral and when superficial may be slightly mobile, usually soft to firm, slowly enlarging over years. Malignant: firm to hard, fixed, rapid growth over a number of months, facial nerve involvement and infiltration of surrounding tissues.

13. Facial nerve injury (which may be unavoidable in treating malignant disease), Frey's syndrome, gustatory sweating due to divided parasymphathetic nerves growing into the skin, salivary fistula, recurrence of malignancy.

CHAPTER 8: THE BREAST

1. A focal area of lobular stromal hyperplasia with epithelial proliferation.

2. Non-cyclical breast discomfort with or without swelling or nodularity. When present, nodularity may be both palpable and tender and may include cystic changes.

3. Fibroadenoma, fibroadenosis, acute and chronic infection, fat necrosis, sclerosing adenonis, granulomatous lobular and periductal mastitis, and eczematous disease of the nipple.

4. Mammography screening of the female population at age 51 to 70 may detect non-palpable asymptomatic disease. Serial assessment at three-year intervals may identify early malignant change. Abnormalities are

detected by specialist teams. When necessary, more precise diagnostic measures are initiated.

5. 80% of symptomatic lesions present with a palpable lump, nipple retraction or a blood strained discharge; axillary mass or Paget's disease are less common; asymptomatic disease may be picked up on screening.

6. Local spread may distort the nipple, tethering to skin may produce peu d'orange and deep tethering may cause fixation. Nodal spread is to the axilla and is frequently to the internal mammary nodes. Vascular spread is primarily to the liver, lung and bone.

7. Paget's disease of the nipple is a sub-epidermoid carcinoma arising in the nipple/areola complex.

8. Bloody discharge from ductal papilloma and carcinoma; green cell debris from fibroadenosis and duct ectasia; yellow exudate from fibroadenosis and abscesses; milk from the lactating breast. Cutaneous discharge may arise from eczematous change.

9/10. Early breast disease is stage 1 (TI: a tumour of < 2cm) and stage 2 (T2: 2–5cm); if axillary nodes are present, they must be mobile. Treatment involves complete local excision of lesions of <5cm as well as radio-therapy to the conserved breast; axillary surgery involves node sampling (four nodes) or axillary clearance below the axillary vein and medial to the pectoralis minor muscle.

11. Lumpectomy conserves breast tissue but requires prophylactic radio-therapy.

12. Advanced cancer is stage III (tumours of >5cm: T3), or extension into the skin or chest wall (T4). Axillary nodes are fixed (N2) and ipsilateral internal mammary nodes are present (N3) and stage 4 extension beyond the breast and chest wall (M1). Treatment involves radiother-apy, endocrine and chemotherapy directed at symptomatic, local and distal sites; these may also be used to downstage locally advanced disease prior to surgery.

CHAPTER 9: THE GASTROINTESTINAL TRACT

1.

Dysphagia may be due to abnormalities of the wall, of the lumen or extrinsic pressure. Strictures of the wall include benign and malignant neoplasms, acute and chronic oesophagitis, Crohn's disease, post-radiotherapy, oesophageal diverticulum and scleroderma. Abnormal contracture occurs in achalasia, abnormal relaxation of the cricopharyngeus and Chargas' disease. Abnormalities within the lumen include foreign bodies and webs. Extrinsic pressure can be from a goitre, pharyngeal pouch, aortic aneurysm or abnormal aortic arch vessels, mediastinal tumours and a paraoesophageal hiatus hernia.

Hepatomegaly: (a) Infection (hepatitis A, B, C, D, E; infectious mononucleosis, hydatid cysts, ameoba, schistosomiasis and bacterial abscesses, cholangitis and portal pyaemia); (b) cellular proliferation (leukaemias, lymphoma, polycythemia); (c) cellular infiltrates (amyloid, sarcoid); (d) metabolic (haemachromatosis, Wilson's disease, galactosemia and drugs); (d) space occupying lesions (abscesses, cysts, syphilitic gumma, haemangioma, hepatoma, colangiocarcinoma, metastatic disease); (e) congestive heart failure and Budd Chiari syndrome.

Splenomegally: (a) Infection (viral, infective mononucleosis, typhoid, thyphus, TB, septicaemic abscess, syphilis, leptospirosis, malaria, schistosomiasis, trypanosomiasis, tropical splenmegally, hydatid cyst and kala-azar); (b) cellular proliferation (leukaemia, myelofibrosis, polycythemia rubra vera, pernicious anaemia, hereditary spherocytosis, thalassaemia, sickle cell disease, idiopathic thrombocytopenic purpura, collagen disease, Felty's disease and syndrome and Still's disease); (c) cellular infiltrates and metabolic (amyloid, Gaucher's disease, porphyria); (d) space occupying lesions (cysts, angiomalymphoma); (e) Circulatory (congestion and portal hypertension, hepatic vein obstruction, right-sided heart failure, embolic infarction, splenic artery infarction and venous thromboses.

Hepatosplemomegally can be determined from the overlap from the previous two lists.

Jaundice may be due to pre-hepatic causes (haemolytic: hereditary spherocytosis, hypersplenism), hepatic causes (liver dysfunction: hepatitis, cirrhosis, Gilbert's disease) and post-hepatic causes (obstruction to the biliary tree due to gallstones, benign and malignant strictures, sclerosing colangiitis, extrinsic neoplasms in the porter hepatis and in the head of the pancreas).

Change in bowel habit: : this is commonly experienced in relation to dietary changes, alcohol intake, overseas trips and changes in daily routines such as mobility, confinement to bed and in pregnancy. However, when there is obvious cause it must be fully investigated since it is a cardinal sign of neoplasia in the older age group, as well as the other pathology listed in the subsequent two items.

Diarrhoea: commonly infective in origin; in temperate climates, salmonella and escherichia are common whereas in tropical areas, a wide variety of bacteria, viral and parasitic agents may be involved. Other causes include: ingestion of purgatives and antibiotics, chronic pancreatitis, cystic fibrosis, small gut abnormalities (e.g, gluten induced or protein losing enteropathy), inflammatory bowel disease (see below), surgical intervention (gastrectomy, vagotomy, blind loop syndrome, small gut resection, stomas), fistulae, and systemic diseases (thyrotoxicosis, uremia, carcinoid and Zollinger's Ellison). Spurious diarrhoea is the leakage of fecal fluid around in impacted faeces.

Constipation is a cardinal sign of acute intestinal obstruction (see below). In these cases there is absolute constipation with no passage of flatus. Other causes include weight loss (starvation cachexia and malignant lesions), peritoneal and inflammatory disorders (appendicitis, pelvic inflammatory disease, peritonitis, perforation), biliary and renal colic, drugs (e.g. analgesics, ganglion blockers), adynamic bowel (Hirschsprung and Chagas'), spinal cord abnormalities, myxoedema, pelvic masses (pregnancy, fibroids, uterine and ovarian tumours), and painful lesions inhibiting defacation (abscesses and complicated haemorrhoids).

Haematemesis and Melaena: Melaena is the name for the black stool resulting from the digestion of blood from luminal bleeding in the upper intestinal tract. When this bleeding is profuse and from the proximal duodenum and above, it may be vomited as haematemesis. Thus, haematemesis and melaena have common etiology above this level. Oesophageal bleeding must be differentiated from haemoptysis and may result from most of the inflammatory and neoplastic causes of dysphagia listed above. Other causes of oesophageal bleeding include trauma following endoscopy, ingestion of foreign bodies and vomiting leading to tearing of the mucosa at the oesophageal junction (Mallory-Weiss tear). Some of the most severe bleeding is from oesophageal varices in liver failure and fatal bleeding occurs when an aortic aneurysm erodes into the oesophagus. Gastroduodenal haematemesis is usually due to peptic ulceration but may be caused by multiple gastric erosions and benign and malignant neoplasms. In the small gut, ectopic gastric mucosa may be present in Meckel's diverticulum or duplicated gut causing melaena. Auto-duodenal fistulae and fistulae from infected prosthetic grafts in the abdomen may also cause malaena.

Bleeding per rectum: may be overt or covert. Covert bleeding is associated with anaemia and usually originates from lesions in the right colon which is more capacious than the left colon and therefore rarely becomes obstructed. The commonest cause of overt bleeding is piles. Other causes include fistulae, fissures and any neoplasm of the colon, rectum or anal canal. Bleeding from inflammatory lesions can be more prominent than from neoplasia. Catastrophic bleeding occasionally occurs from a diverticulum. Although upper alimentary bleeding usually presents as melaena, copious bleeding may pass through the bowel with little such change. Vascular malformations may give rise to severe haemorrhage.

Obstruction: in children may be related to atresia along the length of the gut (oesophageal, pyloric, small gut, Hirschsprung's disease and imperforate anus; duodenum and Ladd's bands, annular pancreas, meconium ileus, mid-gut volvulus, strangulated hernias and intersusception. Adult obstruction may result from adynamic or dynamic causes. Adynamic causes include paralytic ileus, acute ischaemia, megacolon and Hirschsprung's and Chagas' disease and pseudo-obstructoin. Dynamic causes include lesions of the wall, lesions within the lumen and external compression. Lesions within the gut wall include diverticular disease, inflammatory bowel, carcinoma and anastomotic strictures. Luminal obstruction may be due to faecal impaction and gallstone ileus. The most common causes of external compression are adhesions and hernias. Other causes of external compression include volvulus, bands and the spread of neoplasia throughout the peritoneum and pelvis.

Pruritis ani is caused by excess sweating and poor local hygiene, skin conditions (eczema, contact dermatitis, allergy, psoriasis, lichen, planus), infective lesions (sexually transmitted diseases, fungal, scabies, lice, threadworms, candida, trichomonas). Other causes include anal pathology (piles, fissures, fistulae, warts and pilus adenomas, solitary ulcers and other anal neoplasms), diarrhoea/incontinence (sphincter malfunction, rectal prolapse, leakage of liquid paraffin), generalized causes of itching (obstructive jaundice, diabetes mellitus, hypoparathyroidism, myeloproliferative disorders and lymphomas), and psychological causes. In babies, pruritis ani is most commonly due to nappy rash as a result of infrequent changes and reaction to local applications.

2. Abdominal tenderness results from pressure over an area of inflamed parietal peritoneum. Pressure at such sites may produce voluntary contraction (guarding) of the lower abdominal wall. When peritonitis is present (see below), there is involuntary contraction of the muscles producing rigidity. Paradoxically, the board-like rigidity seen in acute pancreatitis and perforated peptic ulcer is not associated with abdominal tenderness, as the wall is too rigid to allow deeper palpitation. When there is deeply-seated or mild inflammation, superficial palpation may not produce tenderness but rapid release from deep palpation produces rebound tenderness. This test, however, must never be performed when tenderness has already been established as it may lead to severe pain. Percussion rebound is a very valuable test as, gently performed, it can localise the point of maximal involvement, such as in childhood appendicitis.

3. Peritonism and peritonitis are signs of peritoneal inflammation and are accompanied by marked guarding and often rigidity. Peritoneal inflammation may results from infective or non-infective causes, leading to peritonitis and peritonism respectively. Uninfected peritonism may be due to leakage of five irritant fluids (gastric and pancreatic juice, bile, urine and blood) due to perforation of a peptic ulcer, gall bladder, acute pancreatitis or bleeding from a ruptured ectopic pregnancy. If left untreated, these conditions progress to acute peritonitis due to secondary infection from transmural migration of gut organisms. Primary blood-borne peritonitis is secondary to bacteria from the lower bowel.

4. Gallstones may present with indigestion. Inflammation may produce tenderness. Impaction of a gallstone in the cystic gut may produce biliary colic or a a mucocoele that may subsequently perforate. Stones in the common bowel duct may produce ascending cholangitis and intermittent or progressive jaundice. They may also erode through into an adjacent small bowel and produce small bowel obstruction.

5. Pancreatic carcinomas are usually slow growing. The symptoms are often vague, deep abdominal or back pain. Diagnosis may be late when they have already invaded adjacent structures, such as the large vessels, spleen and the lesser sac. Carcinomas of the head however, may involve the common bowel duct and investigation of the progressive jaundice results in an earlier diagnosis.

6. Diverticulosis is a common condition in the Western world arising through a diet low in roughage and high in refined foods. Over half the population over the age of 50 are affected. Diverticulitis indicates a superadded infection.

7. Symptoms of diverticular disease include alteration in bowel habit, pain and tenderness in the left iliac fossa, and rectal bleeding which may be severe. Diverticular disease may also present with an abscess and a palpable mass in the left iliac fossa, perforation, peritonitis and sepsis. Fistulae into the bladder produces pneumaturia. Isolated diverticulae in the caecum may present with a mass and be an important differential diagnosis for neoplasia.

8/9. Crohn's disease and ulcerative colitis collectively are termed inflammatory bowel disease and may cause intrinsic or extrinsic lesions. The gut lesions or colitis are primarily ulceration of the mucosa and submucosa of the colon and rectum. Longterm, they are prone to malignant change. Crohn's disease is associated with full-thickness inflammation of the gut wall with fissuring and skip lesions and mainly involves the small bowel but also the large bowel and the perianal region. It typically involves adjacent structures such as the gut, urinary tract, vagina and skin. Ulcerative colitis and is associated with prominent diarrhoea and occasionally fulminating toxic megacolon.

Extra-intestinal manifestation of inflammatory bowel disease include haematological disorders (iron deficieny and haemolytic anaemia, leukocytosis and thrombocytosis and deep vein thrombosis), skin disorders (erythema nodosum, pyodermagangrenosa, drug reactions of erythema multiforme and finger clubbing), ocular disorders (iritis, uveitis, episcleritis, superficial keratitis with blepharitis, retinitis, retrobulbar neuritis), hepatic disease (sclerosing chlonangitis, perichlangitis, fatty infiltration, cholelithiasis), renal disease (immune mediated pyelonephritis, nephrolithiasis, glomerulin nephritis, hypokalemic nephritis) and arthropathy (ankylosing spondylitis, sacroilitiis, migratory monoarthropathy, peripheral arthritis in children).

10. Duke's A: neoplasmic confined to gut wall; Duke's B: spread through gut wall; Duke's C: nodal involvement. Later sub-classifications included C1 and C2 referring to the involvement of nodes around the inferior mesenteric artery, and D for metastatic spread.

11. Lesions of the capacious right colon where faecal material is more fluid, usually present with anaemia. Lesions of the left colon may present with an alternation in bowel habit and/or obstruction. Both may present with a palpable mass or spread to the adjacent peritoneum leading to an inflammatory mass or perforation. Both may also present with signs of secondary spread to the liver.

12. The features of intestinal of obstruction are colicky abdominal pain, vomiting, abdominal distension and absolute constipation.

13. Extra-abdominal causes of acute abdominal pain are often non-surgical in origin and must always be considered in the differential diagnosis of the acute abdomen. Cardinal signs are the absence of percussion or deep rebound tenderness during abdominal examination. They include ischaemic heart disease, pleuritic irritation from underlying lung disease, somatic nerve and root pain from herpes zoster infection, other causes of spinal root irritation (e.g. degenerative disease of the thoracic spine and tumours and abscesses in the thoracic spinal cord), diabetic crises, hyperparathyroidism, hyperlipidemia, porphyria, lead colic, sickle cell crises, tabes dorsalis and Munchausen's syndrome.

CHAPTER 10: THE GROIN AND SCROTUM

1. A protrusion of the whole or part of a viscus from its normal position, through an opening in the wall of its containing cavity.

2. (a) Lumbar hernia: through a defect in the lateral abdominal wall, above the iliac crest between the posterior border of external oblique

and the anterior border of latissimus dorsi. (b) Umbilical hernia: through a congenital defect in the umbilicus. (c) Paraumbilical hernia: through the linea alba, adjacent to the umbilicus. (d) Incisional hernia: through an old incision. (e) Spigelian hernia: through a defect in the lateral border of the rectus sheath, usually just below the umbilicus. (f) Internal abdominal hernias: through the oesophageal hiatus and other diaphragmatic congenital openings.

3. Indirect: congenital persistence of the processus vaginalis within the spermatic cord and along the inguinal canal into the scrotum. Direct: weakness in the transversalis fascia, below the conjoined tendon, bulging into the posterior aspect of the inguinal canal, medial to the inferior epigastric vessels and passing laterally alongside the spermatic cord through the superficial inguinal ring.

4. The superficial inguinal ring is situated above and medial to the pubic tubercle and is an opening in the external oblique aponeurosis. The deep inguinal ring is situated just above the midpoint of the inguinal ligament and is an opening in the transversalis facia.

5. The inguinal canal extends from the deep to the superficial inguinal rings as described in (4). Posterior relations: the transversalis facia and medially conjoined tendon and inferior epigastric vessels passing upwards and medially on the tranversalis facia. Anterior relations: the external oblique and laterally the internal oblique. Inferior relations: the inguinal ligament and medially the lacunar reflection of the inguinal ligament. The internal oblique arches over the canal to become the conjoined tendon.

6. The neck of femoral canal is situated lateral to the lacunar ligament, medial to the femoral vein, with the inguinal ligament anteriorly and the superior pubic ramus posteriorly. The canal passes downwards beneath the fascia lata to the saphenous opening. Hernias passing along this pathway and through the opening alongside the vein. Because of the attachment of the superficial facia to the inferior margin of the saphenous opening, femoral hernias then are directed upwards anterior to the inguinal ligament in the groin.

7/8. Two serious complications of hernias are obstruction and strangulation. In obstruction, constriction of the neck of the sac leads to obstruction of the loops of small bowel within it. In strangulation, constriction of the venous return leads to congestion, arterial occlusion and gangrene, with the potential of perforation causing peritonitis or a groin abscess. In a Richter's hernia, a bulge of one wall of the viscus into the hernial sac may become strangulated without producing obstruction of the involved bowel loop.

9. An indirect hernia passes along the inguinal canal within the spermatic cord and its congenital defect. A direct inguinal hernia is through a weakness of the transversalis facia in the posterior wall, the hernial sac passing medially through the superficial inguinal ring alongside the spermatic cord.

10. Herniotomy involves the opening of the hernial sac, the inspection of its contents, their replacement within the abdominal wall, ligation of the neck and the removal of excess tissues. In herniorrhaphy, there is additional repair of the abdominal wall defect. In children, where the superficial and deep inguinal rings almost overlap, a herniorrhaphy is unnecessary as, in the subsequent development of the inguinal canal, the external and internal oblique muscles come to overlie the herniotomy site.

11. An incision is made over the strangulated loop of gut, the sac is opened, infected peritoneal fluid is evacuated, and the strangulated loop is examined to assess its viability and the need for resection. Care must be taken not to lose a strangulated loop or strangulated side wall of bowel back into the abdomen without it being fully examined. If there is any doubt about this happening, or if the resection cannot be carried out through the hernial sac, a separate laparotomy incision is also required.

12. The initial diagnosis is a clinical one. Tumour markers may be elevated: beta human chorionic gonadotropin (90% in teratoma, 25% seminoma), alpha feta protein (50% in teratoma) and alkaline phosphatase (50% in seminoma). CT identifies para-aortic or mediastinal lymph nodes or secondaries in the liver or lungs. The treatment is orchidectomy via an inguinal approach. The testes is delivered through the incision in the external oblique and a vascular clamp is applied to the spermatic cord whilst a biopsy and frozen section are taken to confirm the diagnosis. A high ligation of the cord and orchidectomy are then undertaken. Subsequent management depends on the stage and the pathology. Stage I: rising tumour markers postorchidectomy; stage 2: abdominal nodes; stage 3: supradiaphragmatic nodes; stage 4: lung or liver metastases.

Treatment of seminomas: radiotherapy for stages 1 and 2. Combination chemotherapy for stage 2 if nodes are greater than 5cm and for cysts after radiotherapy, and for stages 3 and 4. Treatment of teratomas: surgical resection of abdominal nodes as well as combination chemotherapy. Treatment of lymphomas: orchidectomy and chemotherapy.

CHAPTER 11: ARTERIAL INSUFFICIENCY OF THE LOWER LIMB

1. The blood supply is insufficient to keep the tissues alive; ischaemic metabolites and associate ulceration produce pain.

2. Turbulence when blood encounters a narrowing. High flow (associated with arteriovenous fistulae) may produce a bruit or a continuous murmur (machinery murmur). Murmurs may be transmitted from the heart, particularly to the carotid vessels.

3. (a) The effect on lifestyle: how far they can and need to walk, interference with work activities and social life; (b) response to preventative measures, e.g. stopping smoking, reaching an optimal weight and regular exercise; (c) the rate of progress.

4. In diabetes, arterial disease occurs a decade earlier than in the rest of the population and is complicated by microvascular disease, neuropathy of motor or sensory and autonomic fibres, and increased susceptibility to infection.

5. Early onset of arteriosclerotics occurs in hyperlipidemia, antiphospholipid syndrome, a bad family history, diabetes, a heavy smoker and Beurger's disease. Also consider compartment syndromes, popliteal entrapment and cystic degeneration, arterial injury, congenital anomalies and exclude pain of neurological origin.

6. Trauma, embolism and thrombosis of aneurysms or pre-existing chronic disease.

7. The six P's: pain, paraesthesia, paralysis, pallor, pulselessness, perishingly cold.

8. The ABPI is the ratio of the ankle to the arm blood pressure – usually over 1 since the muscle bulk of the leg gives slightly higher readings. The value is reduced in lower limb arterial disease with a further fall of exercise.

9. Leg disease commonly starts in the superficial femoral artery at the adductor hiatus, or its origin. Symptoms become prominent once disease is present at two levels, such as with additional popliteal or aorto-iliac stenosis.

10. Family history, hyperlipidemia, diabetes, smoking and hypertension.

CHAPTER 12: VENOUS DISORDERS OF THE LOWER LIMB

1. Varicose veins are superficial, thin walled, elongated, tortuous dilated veins. They may be primary congenital in origin when there is often a family history. Both primary and secondary varicose veins are associated with valvular incompetence of the superficial system. Secondary varicose veins are associated with disease of the deep veins, e.g. previous deep vein thrombosis giving rise to superficial venous hypertension. Varicose veins may also be associated with arteriovenous malformations and fistulae.

2. Venous insufficiency describes a failure of the normal venous circulation: valves direct blood from the superficial to the deep vessels and from there, propelled by muscle pumps, back to the heart. It is associated with venous hypertension causing swelling and aching of the legs, particularly at the end of the day, and progressive skin changes – eczema, pigmentation, bleeding thrombosis, lipodermatosclerosis and ulceration.

3. Injection and/or surgery are indicated when the cosmetic appearance or the discomfort of the primary veins or their complications are unacceptable to the patient.

4. There are no symptoms in 50% of patients with deep venous thrombosis. The commonest symptoms are a pale, swollen lower leg, calf tenderness and pain on active and passive plantar and dorsiflexion. If thrombosis extends enough to impair venous return, a blue swollen leg can lead to necrosis of superficial tissues; venous gangrene has a 50% amputation rate.

5. Thrombosis is produced by damage to the vessel wall, stasis and alteration in the constituents of the blood. These are all present after surgery and also when the patient is confined to bed. Hormonal changes also predispose to deep vein thrombosis, e.g. in association with the oral

contraceptive pill, pregnancy, puerperium, hormonal replacement therapy. Thrombophlebitis is associated with serious illness, particularly malignancy.

6.   Venous gangrene, pulmonary embolism and late sequele of long term venous insufficiency.

CHAPTER 13: THE HIP

1.   Congenital dislocation of the hip occurs in up to 20/1000 live deliveries. It has a polygenic inheritence pattern and is associated with high maternal hormones and breach position of the baby. It is associated with acetabular and proximal femoral dysplasia.

2.   In neonates, screen with Ortolani's test: abduction of the hips in 90° flexion is impeded; pressure on greater trochanters reduces the hips with a clunk and further movement is then possible. Barlow's test attempts to lever the hips in and out of the acetabulum during abduction. Late features are asymmetry, clicking, and difficulty in changing nappies.

3.   Diagnosis by clinical tests, ultrasound. After six months, X-rays: look for Von Rosen's line (45° abduction line is drawn through femoral shaft and should point to the acetabulum) and Perkin's line (femoral head epiphysis should lie below a horizontal line through the triradiate cartilage, medial to the vertical line drawn from the outer acetabular edge). Treatment: 3–6 months, double nappies for six weeks; 6 months: abduction splint. If still unstable, 6–18 months: traction, plaster spica or open surgery. If unsuccessful, 18 months- 10 years: traction followed by surgery and 3 months hip spica. Treatment after this time, or after 6 years in bilateral cases, should be avoided during development to prevent avascular necrosis of femoral head.

4.   A slipped upper femoral epiphysis is a posterior displacement of the upper femoral epiphysis, usually in boys age 14–16 years who are overweight or tall and thin. Due to hormonal imbalance and trauma, resulting in premature fusion and re-modeling.

5.   Protrusio acetabuli is a pelvic deformity where the medial wall of the acetabulum expands inwards. It is associated with skeletal dysplasias, coxa vara, osteoarthritis, connective tissue disorders, Marfan's syndrome, haemophilia and post-radiotherapy.

6. Perthes' disease is avascular necrosis of the femoral head occurring in boys aged 4–8 years due to post-traumatic joint effusion compressing the lateral epiphyseal vessels. Re-modelling results in an abnormally shaped head.

7. True shortening is due to joint or bony abnormality of the hip, knee or lower leg, and is determined by comparing the distances from the greater trochanter to the lateral malleolus on each side. Apparent shortening is seen when malalignment between the ankles (on lying) is produced by pelvic tilting, as occurs in a fixed adduction deformity. Measurement from the umbilicus or symphysis pubis highlights the difference on two sides.

8. **Osteoarthritis**: asymmetric narrowing of the joint space with sclerosis of subcondylar bone, cysts close to the joint surface and osteophytes at the joint margin. **Rheumatoid arthritis**: periarticular osteoporosis, marginal bony erosion, narrowing of joint space. At later stages, destruction and deformity, with subluxation of the joint surfaces.

9/10. Analgesia: Paracetamol is preferred to longterm nonsteroidal antiinflammatory drugs. Physiotherapy and the use of a walking stick reduce weight bearing. With progressive pain and limitation in mobility and activity, surgery is considered. Initially a subtrochanteric osteotomy but, in late cases, an arthrodesis or a prosthetic joint replacement may be required.

11. (a) Chronic infection with pain and wound sinuses, affecting 1% of hip replacements. X-rays show changes in areas around implant. Requires removal of the prosthesis and replacement with uncemented form. Performed at least four weeks after removal or allowing fibrous pseudoarthrosis to develop. An aseptic lucency may be demonstrated without infection but the pain usually requires prosthetic replacement. (b) Acute dislocation: may require stabilization with a spika after reduction and if recurrent, prosthetic replacement. (c) Heterotopic bone formation producing pain and stiffness: may respond to nonsteroidal antiinflammatory medication.

12. Young patients, particularly those still undertaking active contact sports since any subsequent revision is accompanied by a much higher complication rate; mild disease; severe degenerative disease with destruction of the hip joint or multiple joint involvement; when there is doubt as to the origin of the hip pain such as coexistent scol-

iotic problems; patient refusal or mental apathy towards the procedure; severe comorbidity and obesity.

13. Garden's classification:

- Incomplete impacted fracture.
- Complete undisplaced fracture.
- Moderately displaced fracture.
- Severely displaced fracture.

Displacement disrupts the blood supply of bone, reducing the chances of
natural healing and indicating the need for surgical intervention.

CHAPTER 14: THE KNEE

1. The tibio-femoral angle is 5–7° of femoral valgus. It is usually greater in the female due to the wider pelvis.

2. Genu varum (bow legs): >6cm between the knees when the heels are together. Physiological normal finding in babies; abnormal growth of the posteromedial proximal tibial epiphysis; osteoarthritis and carti-lage loss in the medial compartment; Paget's disease and epiphyseal injury; vitamin C and D deficiency.

3. Genu valgum: >8cm between malleoli with knees touching. Physiological normal variant in toddlers of age 3–4; rheumatoid arthri-tis; dysplasias; epiphyseal injury; vitamin C and D deficiency.

4. Painful swelling of the tibial tubercle in adolescence due to traction injury of the apophysis. Spontaneous recovery with alteration of activ-ity.

5. Avascular necrosis of subchondral bone: avascular fragments separate and may give rise to loose bodies

6. Congenital lesions (e.g. bipartite patella); injuries; stress (growth spurts, chondromalacia patellae, obesity, synovial shelf syndrome); osteochondritis (Osgood-Schlatter's, osteochondritis dissecans); bursae (bursitis, popliteal cysts, Baker's cysts); joint pathology (rheumatoid arthritis, osteoarthritis, tuberculosis).

7. Meniscal tear; loose bodies (joint mice) such as in osteochondritis dissecans; synovial chondromalacia; osteochondral fracture; localized

separation of articular cartilage and plica syndrome (trapping of a synovial fold).

8. Osteoarthritis: asymmetric narrowing of joint space, sclerosis of subcondylar bone; cysts close to the joint surface, and osteophytes at the joint margin.

9. Rheumatoid arthritis: periarticular osteoporosis, marginal bony erosion, narrowing of joint space. At later stages, destruction and deformity, with subluxation of joint surfaces.

10. Splitting is usually along the length of the medial meniscus: bucket handle tears remain attached at each end. It presents with severe pain, usually on the medial side of the knee, often as a sports injury. Occasionally the knee is locked in flexion. Swelling follows a few hours or days later. Recovery is with rest but pain and swelling may recur.

CHAPTER 15: THE HAND AND FOOT

The Hand

1. **Median:** thenar muscles and lateral two lumbricals, flexor digitorum superficialis and lateral two tendons of flexor digitorum profundus. **Ulnar:** hypothenar muscles, adductor pollicis, tendons of flexor digitorum profundus to ring and little finger. **Radial:** lateral forearm muscles (the long extensor tendons are supplied by its posterior intraosseous branch).

2. **Median:** thenar wasting, loss of thumb abduction, flexion of ulnar fingers but pointing of the index finger, loss of wrist flexion and pronation. Loss of sensation over the radial three and a half digits including the nail beds. **Ulnar:** loss of intrinsic muscle function of the hand produces a claw hand with loss of finger abduction and thumb adduction. Loss of sensation over the ulnar one and a half digits including the nail bed. Positive Froment's sign. **Radial:** loss of elbow extension with injuries to the upper arm; loss of extensors of wrist, fingers and thumb, and thumb abduction. Sensory loss over anatomical snuffbox.

3. **Median:** penetrating injuries in the arm and forearm, elbow dislocation, carpal dislocation, carpal tunnel syndrome due to fluid retention in associqation with congestive cardiac failure, pregnancy, connective

tissue disease (rheumatoid arthritis), endocrine disease (acromegally, myxodema).

Ulnar: usually disease around the elbow, e,g. fractures, dislocations, entrapment in the medial epicondular cubital tunnel, particularly with severe valgus deformity and osteoarthritis, compression injuries against the medial epicondyle (during anaesthesia or trauma), penetrating injuries in the forearm, repeated trauma over the posohamate tunnel (in cyclists).

Radial: falling asleep with the arm hanging over the back of a chair (Saturday night palsy), midshaft fracture of the humerus with damage in the spiral groove, penetrating injuries and fracture-dislocation of the elbow.

Prolonged use of a tournique or acute ischaemia can damage all three nerves.

4. Wrist dorsiflex and fingers slightly flexed (as in gripping a tennis ball). A front or backslab is used to retain the hand in this position.

5. de Quervain's is a thickening, inflammation and tenderness of the tendon sheaths of extensor pollicis brevis and longus, and abductor pollicis longus, giving pain on thumb abduction against resistance and passive adduction.

6. Patient's finger clicks when it is bent and usually has to be forcibly straightened. A palpable tendon nodule may be present. Symptoms are due to trapping of the nodule by a stenosis in the sheath.

7. Dupuytren's contracture has an autosomal dominant inheritance, and is associated with alcohol cirrhosis, phenytoin, diabetes mellitus, AIDS and tuberculosis.

The Foot

1. In club foot, the heel is inverted heel, the talus points downwards, the foot is twisted so the foot sole faces posteromedially, and the forefoot is abducted and laterally rotated. The foot cannot be dorsiflexed to touch the leg as is normal in neonates.

2. No treatment required in asymptomatic children or adults. Heel cups or arch supports and physiotherapy may help mild symptoms. Surgery is rarely needed and involves tendon advancement and fusion of the midtarsal metatarsal joints, and excision of prominent bone from the navicular.

3. In hallux valgus, there is excessive lateral angulation of the big toe away from the axis of the metatarsal. It may be treated by appropriate footwear and, when symptomatic (e.g. an infected bunion), the prominent part of the metatarsal head can be excised with a corrective osteotomy. Alternative surgical treatments include excision of the metatarsophalangeal joint or arthrodesis.

4. Hallux rigidus is stiffness of the first metatarsophalangeal joint. Causes include osteoarthritis, trauma, osteochondritis or gout, usually without the associated lateral angulation of the toe of hallux valgus – the gout or the hallux rigidus.

5. Pes cavus is usually idiopathic but may be secondary to neurological disorders such as peroneal muscular atrophy or Friedreich's ataxia. It is often associated with clawing of the toes, with callosities under the metatarsal heads. The metatarsophalangeal joints are extended and the interphalangeal joints are flexed.

CHAPTER 16: THE POST-OPERATIVE PATIENT

1. 2.5–3 litres a day of water; 70 mmol of sodium and 60 mmol of potassium.

2. Fluid loss, (through aspiration via a nasogastric tube, diarrhoea, vomiting, an intestinal fistula and sequestration of fluid into various body cavities) is added to the 2.5–3 litres of daily fluid requirement. However, precise measurement of urine output (a catheter being routinely used after major surgery) is documented on fluid balance charts, also measured losses from other sites. These measurements are supplemented by clinical examination and other tests as described in the response to (3).

3. Signs of dehydration are a rising pulse, falling blood pressure, reduced capillary refill, decreased skin turgor, reduced urine output and falling jugular venous pressure (or central venous pressure when the line is in position). Serial measurement of blood urea and creatinine clearance may show progressive abnormality. Overhydration may be more difficult to diagnose. In a patient with good renal and cardiac function, urine output increases to maintain fluid balance, but, in the elderly, the increased load can give rise to cardiac failure. Signs of fluid overload include peripheral oedema (usually over the sacrum in

recumbent patients or dependent ankle oedema), pulmonary oedema as evidenced by basal creps, dyspnoea and a frothy sputum, pleural effusions, ascities and raised jugular venous pressure. Overload may be due to inappropriate amounts of 5% dextrose and may be associated with hyponatremia.

4. The previous two answers have considered replacing appropriate volume and fluid loss. Attention is also given to the type of fluids prescribed. A typical prescription is 2 litres of 5% dextrose to every litre of dextrose saline to satisfy daily requirements of sodium and carbohydrate. If the fluid loss is through haemorrhage, then this may be replaced by blood transfusion. Attention may also be required to maintaining the circulating osmotic pressure of serum by prescribing a colloid solution, such as haemocel or human albumin. Colloid solutions are less likely than crystalloids to be rapidly excreted by the kidney. The logic of replacing circulating fluid loss with a similar constituent such as human albumin has not been consistently successful.

5. Complications of blood transfusion include acute immunological problems (after transfusing the wrong blood) with ABO and rhesus incompatibility, urticarial and anaphylactic reactions. Other immunological complications include transfusion-related acute lung injury and delayed reactions such as post-transfusion purpura, graft versus host disease and immunomodulatory effects. Non-immunological effects include hypothermia, hyperkalemia, hypercalcemia, congestive cardiac failure, and iron overload. Infection may result from bacterial contamination of the transfusion apparatus or transfer from the donor (e.g. hepatitis B, C, HIV I and II, HTLV I and II, parvovirus, cytomegalovirus, malaria, babesiosis, brucellosis, trypanosomiasis and syphilis).

6. Oliguria is excretion of less than 400ml of fluid over 24 hours.

7. Management of oliguria is dependent on the cause. Post-renal obstructive disease such as prostatic hyperplasia, bladder neck obstruction, stones and tumours must be relieved by catheterisation and appropriate management of the underlying cause. In renal failure, treatment is aimed at avoiding hyperkalemia and retention of waste products. Glucose/potassium solutions may control hyperkalemia but, with progressive disease, haemofiltration or haemodialysis may be required. In pre-renal failure, fluid must be replaced. Rapid infusion may require a wide bore central line, the volume being monitored by

central venous or wedge pressures if a pulmonary artery line is in place. Aliquots of 150ml of fluid can be delivered when the central venous pressure is below 3cmH2O. It may be repeated until the level begins to rise. Other factors of over hydration as described in (3) must also be undertaken to ensure that the reading is not a spurious one and that the quantity of fluid is appropriate.

8. A post-operative increase in pulse rate accompanied by a falling blood pressure indicates inadequate circulating blood volume, due to haemorrhage or fluid loss from other sources. Replacement is urgently required. Crystalloid is prescribed in the acute management and delivered rapidly in monitored aliquots. Blood is considered if haemorrhage is the cause.

9. Venous thrombosis is a common post-operative complication. The thrombotic triad of stasis damage to the vessel wall and alteration of blood constituents are all present. Some degree of calf thrombosis occurs in 50% of patients probably starting at the time of operation, although clinically obvious DVT classically occurs at 7 - 10 days, as does pulmonary embolism. Prophylactic measures are therefore advisable, particularly in prolonged surgery and in high risk groups such as those with previous DVTs, malignancy, obesity and who are over 40. Anti-thrombotic above knee compression stockings are appropriate in all major surgery. Additional prophylactic measures include calf compression devices and subcutaneous heparin 500 iu bd.

10. Fever is defined as >38°C. It is commonly related to infection which may be present in the respiratory and urinary tracts, the uterus, and the skin. Abdominal surgery is particularly associated with peritonitis from leakage of gut flora. Bacteremia may also give rise to cannula infections: particularly susceptible individuals are the young, the old, alcoholics, and patients with cardiac valvular disease, diabetes, and immunosupresion. Non-infective causes of pyrexia include atelectasis, DVT, haemotoma formation, transfusion reactions, myocardial infarction, some tumours (e.g. renal), connective tissue disorders and drug reactions. Malignant hyperthermia is an inherited response to suxamethonium.

11. Pain is an inevitable result of surgery. It may be background, continuous or breakthrough. Milder forms of pain, in patients who can take oral preparations, can be managed with Paracetamol and non-steroidal anti-inflammatory drugs, opioids including codeine, dihy-

drocodeine, oxycodeone and tramadol. For more severe pain, morphia is usually administered; this may be intravenous or intramuscular, or as a continuous possibly patient controlled subcutaneous injection. Local anaesthetic may be injected into wounds at operation and epidural pain control is valuable when appropriate. Enternox is useful for short painful procedures.

12. Wound infection may be inevitable when operating through a contaminated field and is increased if there is haemotoma formation. Organisms may come from the skin, be blood borne or may come from the underlying infective sources, particularly in association with peritonitis.

13. The most common respiratory complication is infection. Dry gasses and reduced ciliary movement produce debris and, together with oropharyngeal secretions, this predisposes towards tracheobronchitis, pneumonia and acute respiratory distress syndrome. Atelectasis is also common as ventilation is not uniform throughout the pulmonary tree under anaesthesia, and the debris causing infection also may block bronchi and bronchioles. Reduced post-operative ventilation may be due to diaphragmatic splinting and sedation, and is increased in smokers and patients with previous respiratory problems. Pneuomothorax may be due to hyperinflation and misplaced central lines. Pulmonary embolism may follow a DVT.

14. Diabetics undergoing major surgery should be brought into hospital two to three days pre-operatively. Type I patients should be converted to short acting insulin. In type II, oral medication should be changed to a short-acting sulphonylurea. On the day of the operation, an insulin glucose infusion should be commenced. The concentrations will depend on the patient's expected requirement but typically 15 units in a 500ml pack of 5% dextrose can deliver 3 units in 100ml aliquot delivered over an hour. Concentrations are varied with hourly blood sugar estimations and potassium supplement may be added to the infusion.

Recommended reading list

GENERAL SURGICAL TEXTS

Essential Surgery. Problems, diagnosis and management.
Burkitt H G, 3rd edition, Churchill Livingstone 2001.
A popular textbook of general surgery aimed at clinical medical students. Its main advantages are its very readable style, clear explanations of the pathophysiological basis of surgical problems and illustrated synopses of the main stages of common surgical operations.

Lecture Notes in General Surgery.
Ellis H and Calne R, 10th edition, Blackwell Scientific 2002.
In this text, each surgical disease is consistently classified with useful sections on pathology and management. This is especially helpful for knowing how to structure essay questions.

Surgical Diagnosis and Management: A Guide to General Surgical Care.
Dunn D C and Rawlinson J N, 2nd edition, Blackwell Scientific 1991.
This well-structured text strikes a balance between explaining general principles and giving practical details for the day-to-day management of surgical patients (eg when drains and sutures come out). It will be particularly useful on the wards in the final year and during house jobs.

An Introduction to the Symptoms and Signs of Surgical Disease.
Browse N, 2nd edition, Edward Arnold 1991.
This is a very thorough guide to surgical examination technique and differential diagnosis of common signs. It is very useful for reference but you may find a smaller, more concise guide more practical for carrying about on the wards.

Clinical Examination of the Patient.
Lumley J S P and Bouloux P M G, Butterworth Heinemann 1994.
This pocket reference book, illustrated with 468 colour photographs, serves as a useful guide for formulating and perfecting your clinical examination technique for finals.

Bailey and Love's New Short Practice of Surgery.
Mann C V, Russell R C G, Williams N S, Bulstrode C J K, 23rd edition, Hodder Arnold 2000.
A complete reference surgical textbook if you are unsure of a particular point.

Spot Diagnosis in General Surgery.
Ellis H, 2nd edition, Blackwell Scientific 1993.
A collection of colour photographs of patients, pathology specimens and X-rays. Each photograph is accompanied by background information and relevant questions. A useful revision aid for the short cases and viva.

Oxford Handbook of Clinical Surgery.
McLatchie G R, Oxford University Press 2001.
This pocket handbook is useful for carrying about on the wards. It is full of management plans and practical procedures. However there is not much explanation of basic principles and, while structured, the format is not consistent. It should not be mistaken for a basic surgical text.

Pocket Examiner in Surgery.
Northover J and Treasure T, 2nd edition, Churchill Livingstone 1996.
This pocket book is full of questions and answers and is very useful for carrying around on the wards and quizzing each other when bored or waiting for teaching.

ORTHOPAEDIC TEXTS

Concise System of Orthopaedics and Fractures.
Apley A G and Solomon L, 2nd edition, Butterworth Heinemann 1994.
A popular basic orthopaedics book, full of useful sketches, photographs and X-rays which bring the text to life. Includes examination schemes for different joints.

Clinical Orthopaedic Examination.
McRae R, 4th edition, Churchill Livingstone 1997.
A very thorough guide to examining orthopaedic cases. Each step in the examination schemes is clearly illustrated with a line drawing. Reading this textbook is the nearest you will get to being taught at the bedside.

Physical Signs in Orthopaedics.
Klenerman L and Walsh H J, BMJ Publishing Group 1994.
Over 200 black and white photographs with questions and answers. A useful revision aid, particularly for spot diagnoses in the short cases.

Revision index

abdomen 72–88, 177–82
amputation 115
anatomy 18
  femoral canal 98, 183
  inguinal canal 94–6, 183
  lower limb vasculature 112, 121–2
aneurysm
  aortic 74, 83, 84, 115
  femoral 99
  popliteal 148
ankle 171
ankle-brachial pressure index (ABPI) 185
antalgic gait 133
anterior tibial compartment syndrome 111
anterior triangle of neck 43, 52, 173–4
aortic aneurysm 74, 83, 84, 115
aorto-iliac disease 113, 132
appendix 85
apprehension test 141
arm, examination 169, 171
arterial disease 105–16, 185–6
arterial ulcer 36, 38
arterio-venous (AV) malformations 124
arthritis
  hand 158–9, 159–60
  hip 111, 133, 134–5, 136, 187
  knee 144–5, 146, 147, 189
arthroplasty (hip) 136
ascites 74, 87

Baker's cyst 148
basal cell carcinoma 38, 173
beer-bottle leg 123
bladder 86
blood transfusions 193
boils 34, 173
Boutonniere's deformity 158
bow legs 146, 189
bowel habits 69, 177–9
branchial cyst 52, 56–7
breast 59–68, 175–6
bruit 184
Buerger's test 109, 114
bulge test 139
bunions 161, 192
bursitis 146–8

caecum 84
calculi
  gallstones 181
  salivary gland 58, 175
carbuncles 34, 173
carcinoma
  basal cell 38, 173
  breast 63–5, 66, 67, 68, 175–6
  caecum 84
  colon 85–6, 181
  pancreas 83, 84, 181
  squamous cell 38, 39, 173
  stomach 83
  thyroid 50, 174
carotid body tumour 52, 56
carpal tunnel syndrome 154, 156

cauda equina claudication 111
cervical lymphadenopathy 41,
    46–7, 52–3, 58, 173
cervical rib 56, 157, 160
claudication 110–13, 116, 185
claw toe 161, 192
clawed hand 157–8
clergyman's knee 147
club foot 191
colloid 168, 193–4
colon 84, 85–6, 179, 181–2
colostomy 77
compressibility 27, 99
constipation 69, 87, 178
contracted hand 155–6, 191
cough impulse 92, 99, 100, 119
Courvoisier's law 82
Crohn's disease 85, 181–2
crystalloid 168, 193–4
cysts
    branchial 56–7
    dermoid 35
    epididymal 103
    knee 148
    renal 81
    sebaceous 33
    thyroglossal 43, 52

de Quervain's tenosynovitis 154,
    191
deep venous insufficiency 37, 123
deep venous thrombosis (DVT)
    121, 125, 186–7, 194
dehydration 192
dermatofibroma 31
dermoid cyst 35
diabetes

diabetic foot 114, 185
    operative management 195
diarrhoea 69, 87, 178
direct hernia 90, 96–7, 183, 184
disc prolapse 132, 133
dislocation of hip 136, 187
distension of abdomen 87
diverticulae, knee 148
diverticular disease 85, 181
dorsalis pedis pulse 108
dress code 21–2
dropped finger 158
Dukes' staging 182
Dupuytren's contracture 155–6,
    191
dysphagia 177

eczema 64–5
elbow 157, 171
emergencies 17, 18
epididymal cyst 100, 103
epigastrium 83
Erb's palsy 157
examination techniques 8, 11–12,
    15–16, 21–2
    aortic aneurysm 115
    breast 60–2
    foot 154
    GI tract 70–5, 82, 179
    groin 74, 89–92, 100, 103
    hand 45, 151–4
    hip 127–31, 187
    knee 138–42
    leg 106–10, 117–21, 169–70
    neck 42–8
    post-operative complications
        164–7

swellings 26–8, 42–8
ulcers 29–30
varicose veins 117–21
examiners 3, 16
eye, thyroid disease 41, 45–6

faeces 69, 87, 178–9
femoral aneurysm 99
femoral canal 98, 183
femoral hernia 97–8
femoral pulse 108
femoro-distal disease 113
femur 187, 188, 189
fever 194
fibroadenoma 63, 65, 68, 175
fibroadenosis 63, 66, 67, 68, 175
finger
    Boutonniere's deformity 158
    dropped 158
    mallet 158
    swan neck deformity 159
    trigger 159, 191
Finkelstein's test 154
fistula 57
fixation 61, 64
flat foot 162, 191
flatus 87
fluid balance 192–3
fluid thrill 27–8, 74, 87
foot 154, 161, 162, 191–2
    diabetic 114, 185
Frey's syndrome 175
Froment's sign 154
furuncles 34, 173

gait
    abnormalities in 133–4

claudication 110–13, 116, 185
    examination of 105, 127, 131,
        138
gallbladder 82, 84
gallstones 181
ganglion 35–6
Garden's classification 189
gastric carcinoma 83
gastrointestinal (GI) tract 69–88,
        177–82
    post-operative symptoms 163–4
genitalia *see* testis
genu valgum 146, 189
genu varum 146, 189
goitre 41, 42, 43–6, 49–51
Graves' disease 51
groin 74, 89–104, 182–5
gummatous ulcer 37

haemangioma 32, 34–5
haematemesis 178–9
hallux rigidus 192
hallux valgus 161, 192
hammer toe 161
hand 45, 151–60, 162, 190–1
Hashimoto's thyroiditis 50, 51
hepatomegaly 73, 78, 84, 177
hepatosplenomegaly 80, 177
hernia 89–98, 104, 182, 183, 184
herniorrhaphy 97, 184
herniotomy 97, 184
hip 111, 127–36, 171, 187–9
histiocytoma 31
history-taking 7–8
    amputation 115
    breast 59
    GI tract 69

groin 89
hand 151
hip 127
knee 137
leg 105–6, 115, 117
pain 25, 105, 127, 137
post-operative complications
   163–4
swellings 25, 41
thyroid status 41–2
Horner's syndrome 157
housemaid's knee 147
hydradenitis suppurativa 34
hydrocoele 100, 101–3
hypersplenism 79
hyperthyroidism 41–2, 44–6, 51,
   58, 174
hypertrophic scar 32, 173
hypochondrial areas 82, 83–4
hypothyroidism 42, 44–6, 51, 174

ileostomy 77
iliac fossae 84–6
indirect hernia 90, 96–7, 183,
   184
infective ulcer 36, 38
inflammatory bowel disease 85–6,
   181–2
inguinal canal 94–6, 183
inguinal swellings 89–99, 104,
   183, 184
inguinoscrotal swellings 100–3
intermittent claudication 110–13,
   116, 185
ischaemia
   acute 110, 116, 185–6
   critical 114, 116, 185

pain 132
ulcers 36, 37

jaundice 76, 177–8
joint mice 145
joints, examination 171

keloid scar 32, 173
keratin horn 33
keratoacanthoma 33
keratosis, seborrhoeic 30
kidney 73, 80–1, 83, 84
Klumpke's palsy 157–8
knee 132, 137–49, 171, 189–90
knock knees 146, 189

leg *see* lower limb
Leriche's syndrome 113
ligaments 140–1, 145
lipoma 35
liver 70, 73, 78, 80, 83, 84, 177–8
locking (knee) 137, 145, 149,
   188
loins 84
long cases
   format ix-x, 3, 7–9
   lower limb examination 106,
      108, 127, 128
long saphenous vein 121
lower limb
   arterial disease 105–16, 185–6
   examination 169–70, 171
   foot 154, 161, 162, 191–2
   hip 111, 127–36, 187–9
   knee 132, 137–49, 189–90
   venous disease 117–25, 186–7,
      194

lumps
  general examination 26–8, 39,
    173
  history 25
  see also breast; groin; neck; skin
lymphadenopathy
  cervical 41, 46–7, 52–3, 58, 173
  inguinal 99

malignant melanoma 31, 39, 173
mallet finger 158
mammography 68, 175
McMurray's test 141
median nerve 153, 156, 160, 190
melaena 178–9
melanoma 31, 39, 173
meniscus 141, 145, 189–90
menstrual cycle 59, 66
meralgia paraesthetica 132, 133
molluscum sebaceum 33
myxoedema 51

naevus
  pigmented 31, 39, 173
  strawberry 34–5
neck 41–58, 173–5
neoplastic ulcer 36, 38
neuropathic ulcer 36, 37
nipple
  abnormalities 64–5
  discharge 59, 66–7, 176
Nottingham Prognostic Index 65

obstruction (intestinal) 89, 94, 179,
    181
oesophagus 176, 178–9
oligouria 193

orchidectomy 101, 185–6
OSCEs
  format x-xi, 11–13
  lower limb examination 107,
    128
Osgood-Schlatter's disease 147,
    149, 189
OSLERs
  format ix-x, 3, 7–9
  lower limb examination 106,
    108, 127, 128
osteoarthritis
  hand 160
  hip 111, 133, 134–5, 136,
    187
  knee 144–5, 146, 189
osteochondritis dissecans 149,
    189
ovary 86
overhydration 192, 193

Paget's disease 64–5, 176
pain
  abdominal 70, 72, 180, 182
  claudication 110, 111
  hip 127, 131–3, 134
  history 25, 105
  knee 137, 142–6, 149, 189
  post-operative 163, 194–5
  rest pain 114, 116, 185
pancreas 83, 84, 181
panic, avoidance of 15–16, 22
papilloma 30
parotid gland 48, 52, 54–6, 58,
    174–5
patella 139, 141, 143, 147
pathology specimens 18

patients
    attitude towards 7, 11, 60, 70
    characteristics of x, 3–4
pelvis 187
perforator veins 119–20, 122, 123
peripheral vascular system
    arterial 105–16, 185–6
    venous 117–25, 186–7
peritonism 180
peritonitis 180, 181
Perthes' disease 188
Perthes' test 120
pes cavus 161, 192
pes planus 162, 191
Phalen's test 154
pigmented naevus 31, 39, 173
polycystic kidney 81
popliteal aneurysm 148
popliteal cyst 148
popliteal pulse 108
port wine stain 35
post-operative complications
    163–8, 192–5
posterior tibial pulse 108
posterior triangle of neck 43, 52
potassium 191
pregnancy 86, 87
presentation to examiners 9
protrusio acetabuli 187
pruritis ani 180
psoas abscess 99
pulsatility 27, 115
pulses 108, 115
pyogenic granuloma 32
pyrexia 194

radial nerve 153, 157, 190, 191

rectal bleeding 179
reducibility 27
renal disease *see* kidney
respiratory system, post-operative
    symptoms 163, 195
rest pain 114, 116, 185
revision for the exam 4–5
rheumatoid arthritis
    hand 158–9, 159–60
    hip 187
    knee 144–5, 147, 189
Richter's hernia 94, 98, 184
rodent ulcer 38, 173

sacroiliac pain 132
salivary glands 48, 52, 54–6, 58,
    174–5
saphena varix 99
saphenous veins 121–2
scars 32, 173
    abdominal 76
sciatica 111
scrotum 90–1, 100–3
sebaceous cyst 33
seborrhoeic keratosis 30
senile warts 30
short cases
    format x-xi, 11–13
    lower limb examination 107,
    128
short saphenous vein 122
shortening of the leg 129, 134–5,
    188
shoulder 171
sialoadenitis 54
sieves 16
sinus 57

skin
lumps 30–8, 173
venous insufficiency 123
skin tag 30
small bowel 84, 85, 178, 179,
180–2
sodium 192
spermatocoele 100, 103
splenomegaly 73, 79–80, 81, 83,
84, 177
squamous cell carcinoma 38, 39,
173
squamous cell papilloma 30
staging of cancer
breast 65, 176
colorectal 181
testicular 101, 184–5
stenosing tenosynovitis 159
stomach 83, 178
stomas 77
stools 69, 87, 178–9
strangulation (hernia) 89, 94, 184
strawberry naevus 34–5
submandibular gland 48, 52, 54–5,
58, 174–5
superficial venous insufficiency
123
suprapubic masses 86
swan neck deformity 159
sweat gland infections 34
swellings
general examination 26–8, 39,
173
history 25
see also breast; groin; neck;
skin
syphilis 37

talipes (club foot) 191
tap test 119
tenderness, abdominal 72, 180
tenosynovitis
de Quervain's 154, 191
stenosing 159
testis 90–1, 100–3, 184–5
tethering 61, 64
Thomas' test 129–30, 134–5
thrombosis (DVT) 121, 125, 186–7,
194
thyroglossal cyst 43, 52
thyroid disease 41–2, 43–6, 49–51,
58, 174
tibia
compartment syndrome 111
Osgood-Schlatter's disease 147,
149, 189
Tinel's sign 154
toe deformities 161, 162, 192
Tourniquet test 117–18, 119–20
transfusions 193
transillumination 28, 100
traumatic ulcer 36, 37
Trendelenburg test/gait 120, 128,
131, 133–4
trigger finger 159, 191
trochanteric bursitis 132
Troisier's sign 83
tumour markers 100–1, 184

ulcerative colitis 181–2
ulcers 25, 29–30, 36–8, 39, 173
ulnar nerve 153, 154, 157, 160,
190
umbilical region 84
undescended testis 103

upper limb
   examination 169
   hand 151–60, 162, 190–1
urinary system
   bladder 86
   oligouria 193
   post-operative symptoms 164,
      165
uterus 86

varicocoele 101
varicose veins 99, 117–22, 186
vascular disease
   arterial 105–16, 185–6
   venous 117–25, 186–7, 194
venous disease 117–25, 186–7,
   194
venous insufficiency 121, 123,
   125, 186
venous ulcer 36, 37, 38
Virchow's node 83
viva questions 15–19
   arterial disease 116, 185–6
   breast 68, 175–6
   foot 162, 191–2
   GI tract 88, 177–82

groin 104, 182–5
hand 162, 190–91
hip 136, 187–89
knee 149, 189–90
lumps and ulcers 39, 173
neck and thyroid 58, 173–5
post-operative complications
   168, 192–5
venous disease 125, 186–7
Volkmann's contracture 155,
   156
vomiting blood 178

walking
   abnormalities in 133–4
   claudication 110–13, 116, 185
   examination of 105, 127, 131,
      138
Warthin's tumour 55
warts 30
wasting of hand 160
water requirement 191
wrist
   carpal tunnel syndrome 154,
      156
   examination 171

PASTEST – DEDICATED TO YOUR SUCCESS

PasTest has been publishing books for medical students and doctors for over 30 years. Our extensive experience means that we are always one step ahead when it comes to knowledge of current trends in undergraduate exams.

We use only the best authors, which enables us to tailor our books to meet your revision needs. We incorporate feedback from candidates to ensure that our books are continually improved.

This commitment to quality ensures that students who buy PasTest books achieve successful exam results.

Delivery to your door
With a busy lifestyle, nobody enjoys walking to the shops for something that may or may not be in stock. Let us take the hassle and deliver direct to your door. We will dispatch your book within 24 hours of receiving your order.

How to Order:
www.pastest.co.uk
To order books safely and securely online, shop at our website.

Telephone: +44 (0)1565 752000 Fax: +44 (0)1565 650264
For priority mail order and have your credit card to hand when you call.

Write to us at:
PasTest Ltd
FREEPOST
Haig Road
Parkgate Industrial Estate
Knutsford
WA16 7BR

PASTEST BOOKS FOR MEDICAL STUDENTS

PasTest are the specialists in study guides and revision courses for medical qualifications. For over 30 years we have been helping doctors to achieve their potential. The PasTest range of books for medical students includes:

EMQs for Medical Students Volume 1   1 901198 65 0
EMQs for Medical Students Volume 2   1 901198 69 3
Adam Feather et al

Essential MCQs for Medical Finals, Second edition   1 901198 20 0
Rema Wasan, Delilah Hassanally, Balvinder Wasan

Essential MCQs for Surgical Finals, Second edition   1 901198 15 4
Delilah Hassanally, Rema Wasan

Essential MCQs in Clinical Pharmacology   1 901198 32 4
Delilah Hassanally, Rema Singh

Essential MCQs in Obstetrics and Gynaecology   1 901198 34 0
Diana Hamilton-Fairley

OSCEs for Medical Undergraduates, Volume 1   1 901198 04 9
Adam Feather, Ramanathan Visvanathan, John SP Lumley

OSCEs for Medical Undergraduates, Volume 2   1 901198 05 7
Ramanathan Visvananthan, Adam Feather, John SP Lumley

Medical Finals: Passing the Clinical   0 906896 43 6
Christopher Moore, Anne Richardson

Medical Finals: Structured Answers and Essay Questions   0 906896 79 7
Adam Feather, Ramanathan Visvanathan, John SP Lumley

Surgical Finals: Structured Answers and Essay Questions, Second Edition   1 901198 43 X
Ramanathan Visvanathan, John SP Lumley

Learning by Lists for Medical Students   1 901198 30 8
Stuart McPherson

The Practical Guide to Medical Ethics and Law for Junior Doctors and Medical Students   1 901198 76 6
Chloe-Maryse Baxter, Mark Brennan, Yvette Coldicott

Radiology Casebook for Medical Students   1 901198 40 5
Rema Wasan, Alan Grundy, Richard Beese

Clinical Skills for Medical Students: A Hands-on Guide   1 901198 86 3
Ian Bickle, David McCluskey, Barry Kelly